NATIONAL INSTITUTE SOCIAL SERVICES LIBRARY

Vol

T0256331

VOLUNTEERS IN PRISON AFTER-CARE

VOLUNTEERS IN PRISON AFTER-CARE

AFTER-CARE

The Report of the Teamwork Associates
Pilot Project

HUGH BARR

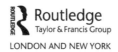

Routledge
Taylor & Francis Group

LONDON AND NEW YORK

First published in 1971 by George Allen & Unwin Ltd

This edition first published in 2022
by Routledge
4 Park Square, Milton Park, Abingdon, Oxon OX14 4RN
605 Third Avenue, New York, NY 10017

Routledge is an imprint of the Taylor & Francis Group, an informa business

British Library Cataloguing in Publication Data
A catalogue record for this book is available from the British Library

ISBN: 978-1-03-203381-5 (Set)
ISBN: 978-1-00-321681-0 (Set) (ebk)
ISBN: 978-1-03-204162-9 (Volume 3) (hbk)
ISBN: 978-1-03-204170-4 (Volume 3) (pbk)
ISBN: 978-1-00-319079-0 (Volume 3) (ebk)

DOI: 10.4324/9781003190790

Publisher's Note
The publisher has gone to great lengths to ensure the quality of this reprint but points out that some imperfections in the original copies may be apparent.

Disclaimer
The publisher has made every effort to trace copyright holders and would welcome correspondence from those they have been unable to trace.

VOLUNTEERS IN PRISON AFTER-CARE

THE REPORT OF THE TEAMWORK ASSOCIATES
PILOT PROJECT

HUGH BARR

WITH A FOREWORD BY
PROFESSOR SIR LEON RADZINOWICZ, LL.D.

London
GEORGE ALLEN & UNWIN LTD
RUSKIN HOUSE MUSEUM STREET

First published in 1971

© George Allen & Unwin Ltd, 1971

ISBN 0 04 301032 6

Printed in Great Britain
in 11 point Barbou
by W & J Mackay & Co Ltd
Chatham

'The Secretary of State's view is that, since the main object of after-care is the integration or reintegration of the offender into the community the participation of ordinary members of the community is a necessary part of the process.'

Home Office Circular 238/1965

FOREWORD

by Professor Sir Leon Radzinowicz, LL.D.

———————

This is a book inspired by idealism and the spirit of adventure. But it is notable also for that shrewd assessment of what is practicable, that recognition of what obstacles must be met, that patient readiness to adapt and re-adapt as fresh difficulties or opportunities reveal themselves, which are essential if any adventure is to be realistically undertaken, any ideal transformed into substantial achievement. This is a man writing about something he himself has had a hand in creating. Not that the author and his collaborators have any illusions about how much they have achieved. Theirs was a pilot project, and the interest of their account lies as much in the dead-ends they abandoned as in the paths they have opened up.

Voluntary initiative and voluntary service have long been a most valuable element in English life. In particular, they have played a major part in the care and rehabilitation of prisoners. The tradition must not be allowed to decay, either through lack of enthusiasm from within or lack of encouragement from without. In his opening chapter Mr Barr looks at some of the trends which, though often good in themselves, have threatened this tradition over the past fifty years, and also at some of the compelling reasons which over the past decade have emphasized the need not merely to preserve but to develop it.

The bulk of the book is devoted to a description of the down-to-earth steps that were taken in one area to establish an effective working partnership between professionals and volunteers, the official Probation and After-Care Service and voluntary organizations. To undertake such a task was to bring to light ideological and emotional as well as practical difficulties, and these also are faithfully described and assessed. Instead of generalities about the need for co-operation between all concerned there is a description of the specific kinds of co-operation and of relationships that proved workable and helpful in the London area. Instead of exhortations to 'befriend' released prisoners there is an analysis of the feelings, problems and behaviour of volunteers who have attempted to do so. The traditional approach is not abandoned, but it is subjected at every point to honest scrutiny.

The book is, in one sense, a product of the Cropwood Fellowships, established at the Institute of Criminology by an anonymous benefactor. The Fellowships were designed to give a few of those who spend most of their lives in the hurly-burly of work with offenders a breathing space to read, think and write about some aspect of their work of practical significance to their various services. Mr Barr has used one of these Fellowships to prepare for publication the findings of his pilot study. He recognizes in his Preface the help given him at this stage by two of my colleagues, Miss J. F. S. King and Mr F. H. McClintock. I have no doubt that the book will indeed prove a notable and forthright contribution to the developing partnership between volunteers and the Probation and After-Care Service in the task of restoring offenders. Both practitioners and researchers will agree that it is no more than the beginning of an exceedingly strenuous journey, but it is a beginning very much on the right lines.

Institute of Criminology
University of Cambridge
September 1970

TEAMWORK ASSOCIATES

Sponsors:

M. J. H. Alison, Esq., M.P.
Gordon Bridge, Esq.
The Rt Revd The Lord Bishop of Croydon
The Rt Hon. Lord Justice Edmund Davies
Frank Dawtry, Esq., O.B.E.
S. C. F. Farmer, Esq., O.B.E.
The Hon. Sir Donald Finnemore
The Revd Canon L. Lloyd Rees
George Lowthian, Esq., C.B.E.
The Hon. S. C. Silkin, Q.C., M.P.
The Revd The Lord Soper
The Revd Austen Williams
The Most Revd The Archbishop of York

Committee:

D. H. Thornton, Esq. (Chairman)
J. H. Fitch, Esq. (co-opted 11 December 1967)
D. L. Griffiths, Esq. (resigned 5 June 1968)
The Revd J. B. Harrison (Company Secretary)
The Revd J. A. Hoyles (co-opted 18 November 1967)
R. K. Nuttall, Esq.
The Revd K. S. Pound (co-opted 11 September 1968)
E. G. Pratt, Esq.
The Revd B. D. Reed
D. D. Sellon, Esq.
F. M. Thomas, Esq. (co-opted 11 September 1968)
E. A. Towndrow, Esq. (co-opted 10 July 1967)
H. J. Wilkinson, Esq. (resigned 14 June 1967)

ACKNOWLEDGEMENTS

The kind of project described in this report is a collaborative effort by hundreds of people. It would be impossible to acknowledge each; nor would they wish it.

I am, however, indebted to committee members, voluntary associates, probation officers and others for their contribution to the project, and for their personal support and encouragement. In particular, I wish to record my thanks to Mr D. H. Thornton (Chairman of the project) and to Mr S. C. F. Farmer (then Principal Probation Officer for Inner London) and his senior staff, without whose consistent interest and support the project would not have been possible.

A special note of appreciation is due to those who backed the project financially, including: the Sir Halley Stewart Trust, the Rowntree Social Service Trust, the Goldsmiths Company, and the Inner London Probation and After-Care Committee.

I am grateful to Professor Sir Leon Radzinowicz, Director of the Institute of Criminology at the University of Cambridge, for the opportunity to prepare this report as one of the Cropwood Fellows, and to the staff of the Institute, particularly my advisers, Mr F. H. McClintock and Miss J. F. S. King, for their help and constructive criticism.

Thanks are also due to Mr R. L. Morrison and Mr Robin Huws Jones, who commented on the text; to Miss L. J. Wilson, my personal assistant during the project, who helped to collect data for the report and took over much of the responsibility for my day-to-day work while I was in Cambridge; to those probation officers who provided statistical data or illustrations; to the voluntary associates who completed questionnaires about their work and to those who prepared longer comments.

The Home Office kindly gave permission to quote figures incorporated in Chapter 1.

HUGH BARR

CONTENTS

TABLES

INTRODUCTION

Following a report of the Advisory Council on the Treatment of Offenders in 1963[1] (hereafter referred to as the ACTO Report), prison after-care in England and Wales has been reorganized radically and the first steps have been taken towards the establishment of an effective and comprehensive range of services for the ex-prisoner. The Probation and After-Care Service has greatly extended its after-care functions and also accepted responsibility for prison welfare and, more recently, for those released on parole. Meanwhile voluntary organizations, and individual volunteers, have begun to work out new forms of partnership with the statutory services and to redefine their roles.

Perhaps the most significant trend has been the growing awareness that the Probation and After-Care Service alone and unaided cannot offer the range of provisions needed if the ex-prisoner is to have effective help. Thus, greater efforts must be made to explore ways in which the resources of the community can be mobilized. Many small-scale projects have been launched in various parts of the country under the auspices of either the statutory or the voluntary organizations. One such project is described in this report.

'Teamwork Associates', as it was called, was a pilot project launched in 1966 for a three-year period to explore ways of involving the ordinary citizen in after-care. Based in London, it was an example of how a voluntary organization sought to work in partnership with a statutory service, in this case the Inner London Probation and After-Care Service, and to complement its work. The writer was for two years a member of the working party that set up the project and for three years its director.

The reorganization of after-care cannot be understood in isolation from the wider and more far-reaching changes now beginning throughout the social services. Twenty years after the Beveridge Plan and the spate of post-war social legislation, we have reached a time of critical reappraisal of the whole range of social services. Although the Probation and After-Care Service was outside the terms of reference of the Seebohm Committee its proposals for a broadly based local authority social service are bound to affect the future of probation and after-care. Perhaps even more relevant to this report was the view of the Seebohm Committee[2] on the community as the basis of the 'authority, resources and effectiveness' of the social service. Under the heading 'citizen participation' the Committee expressed its belief 'in the importance of the maximum participation of individuals and groups in the planning, organization and provision of the social services'. It then commented upon the role of volunteers and voluntary organizations.

More recently, the Aves Report[3] on *Voluntary Workers in the Social Services* has illustrated the wide range of help given by volunteers throughout most of the social services. Volunteers in prison after-care must be seen as a small part of the wider voluntary movement, through which the community expresses much of its practical concern for the dependent and the handicapped.

Much of this report is concerned with the contribution of one particular kind of volunteer, namely the 'voluntary associate'. The second Reading Report[4] distinguished between the 'volunteer' and the 'accredited associate' or 'voluntary associate' as we have preferred to call him. That report used 'volunteer' as a generic term 'to mean any volunteer in after-care or other fields of social work', but advised probation officers 'to distinguish between the volunteer who can provide support for a considerable period by a personal relationship', in other words the voluntary associate, 'and the volunteer whose contribution is more likely to be of short duration, in the way of a simple practical task or advice on a technical problem not requiring close personal involvement'. In practice this distinction often becomes blurred, but it is a necessary one if roles are to be defined clearly and so prove a guide when discussing appropriate forms of organization, recruitment, selection, training and supervision.

Although the project was originally designed with the needs of ex-prisoners in mind, in fact voluntary associates were introduced to many individuals who had not been imprisoned and, in some instances, had not been convicted. This poses a problem of terminology in the report. In keeping with professional social-work practice, the word 'client' has been adopted as a generic term, but its appropriateness may be questioned in a non-professional setting. Voluntary associates, themselves, frequently speak of their 'friends', but this too is open to question.

Any report based upon the writer's experience runs a special risk of bias. To minimize this danger, the report was discussed with a cross-section of those involved in the project and the two advisers within the Institute of Criminology offered advice unfettered by direct involvement. At various points in the report reference is made to the opinions of the voluntary associates. Each of the 125 actually engaged in the project in April 1969 was sent a questionnaire and 121 (97 per cent) were returned. (Copies were not sent to those who had withdrawn, nor to those who had only just been accredited for a few weeks.) Copies of the questionnaire and other papers relating to the project have been lodged with the libraries of the following bodies: the National Institute for Social Work Training, the Institute of Criminology, Cambridge, and the Howard League for Penal Reform.

Especially important, of course, is how the client feels about the help extended to him. Unfortunately it has not been possible to study this, other than from occasional comments passed on by voluntary associates or probation officers. Much more attention will need to be given in the future to the opinions of clients in the form of 'market research' to assess the wants and needs of the consumer.

No attempt will be made in this report to compare practice in the United Kingdom with the contribution of volunteers to correctional programmes in foreign countries. It is a major topic which could not be dealt with adequately as a short section of this report. The International Prisoners' Aid Association[5] has prepared a brief but helpful paper surveying the scene in other countries while Stockdale[6] makes reference to volunteers in some continental countries.

A major part of the report deals with matters such as organization and training of voluntary associates but it should not be thought that the client has been forgotten. The development of sound organization and training are prerequisites of effective help. It is through them that there is hope of progress beyond earlier achievements in this field. Thus the interests of the client remains paramount.

REFERENCES

1. *The Organization of After-Care*, A Report of the Advisory Council on the Treatment of Offenders, 1963, HMSO.
2. The Report of the Committee on Local Authority and Allied Personal Social Services, 1968, HMSO.
3. The Report of the Committee on Voluntary Workers in the Social Services, 1969, George Allen & Unwin and the Bedford Square Press.
4. The Place of Voluntary Service in After-Care, Second Report of the Working Party, 1967, HMSO.
5. Ruth and John Baker for the International Prisoners' Aid Association, 'The Role and Potential Value of Volunteers in Social Defence', *International Review of Criminal Policy* No. 24, 1966, United Nations.
6. Eric Stockdale, *The Court and the Offender*, Gollancz 1967, pp. 62-4, 135-6, 185.

———————

CHAPTER 1

THE BACKGROUND TO THE PROJECT

The Pioneers

Throughout history there have always been those ready to help the prisoner or ex-prisoner. The credit for translating isolated acts of compassion into a voluntary movement can be attributed perhaps to the example of the illustrious Elizabeth Fry[1] in the early nineteenth century. It was she who inspired others to visit the prisons—the forerunners of the modern prison visitors and voluntary associates.

Although there were no famous names by which we remember them, volunteers played an active part in the early days of the Probation Service, as well as in the prisons and after-care organizations. The police court missionaries themselves reflected many of the traditions of voluntary service, a factor which was held to justify low remuneration. Some of the early probation officers were volunteers and worked alongside paid staff.

Professionals and Volunteers

But as early as 1914 Leeson[2] wrote of 'professional probation workers' looking 'askance' at the use of voluntary probation officers. A distinction began to be drawn between volunteer probation officers and other volunteers working with probation officers. A report in 1922[3] noted 'a sharp division of opinion' as to the value of the former, but no such misgivings were expressed about the latter. But by 1935 doubts about the contribution of any type of volunteer seemed to be increasing, although opinion was still divided. *A Handbook of Probation*[4] reported unfavourably on several experiments involving volunteers in probation work, but also spoke of 'a vague aversion in many people's minds to the idea that redemptive work should be reserved as the special profession of a class of paid officials'. Although the subsequent 1936 Report[5] echoed earlier reports in encouraging the involvement of volunteers in an auxiliary capacity, it was evident that something had happened among the probation officers themselves which was leading to the exclusion of even these volunteers.

The gradual shift in attitude was clearly associated with the formalization of social casework theory which for a time emphasized the special relationship between 'worker' and 'client' almost to the exclusion of relations with others in the community. This school of thought became dominant by the 1950s and early 1960s and is clearly illustrated in the textbooks of the period (see, for example, Hamilton (1940),[6] Perlman (1957),[7] Biestek (1957)[8]).

Although such theory profoundly influenced training for the major influx of probation officers in the post-war years, its practical effects are more difficult to assess. However, there is some evidence[9] that the new generation of officers emphasized 'one-to-one' interviews in the office setting, with less involvement in their clients' home settings and less use of community resources than did older colleagues.

At the same time efforts to establish a professional identity necessitated a closing of ranks and the exclusion of those who lacked appropriate skills which were associated with training. Thus many unqualified paid workers, as well as volunteers, were left out and their contribution tended to be undervalued.

The Exclusion of the Volunteers

Not surprisingly, many volunteers resented their exclusion, or relegation to seemingly less responsible or less worthwhile tasks, and this helped to engender tension between professionals and volunteers.

In view of these trends it was no surprise that the 1962 Morison Report[10] said that the period since 1936 had 'seen the final and irreversible emergence of the Probation Service as a profession requiring professional training and skill'. Unlike all the earlier reports on the Probation Service it made no reference to volunteers.

The Reintroduction of the Volunteers

But it was the ACTO Report,[11] only a year later, which reopened the whole question of voluntary help. While probation had become professional, after-care had remained in the hands of voluntary bodies, the discharged prisoners' aid societies, which relied heavily upon volunteers. It had long been assumed that ex-prisoners would reject voluntary after-care from an official service. Thus the voluntary societies retained the responsibility despite rising numbers of discharges. With limited funds the number of paid staff was restricted and salaries were inadequate to attract the new professionals. Thus voluntary after-care was largely unaffected by the 'professionalization' of social work.

Many of the after-care volunteers had been involved only in committee work and fund raising, but the 1953 Maxwell Report[12] stimulated fresh efforts to recruit 'voluntary associates' to reinforce the ranks of paid staff in personal work with ex-prisoners. By 1962 Lacey[13] estimated that there were some 450 voluntary associates in England and Wales plus others working informally in 'clusters' with paid workers. He described four schemes launched during the 1950s, two by the Womens Voluntary Service and the others by the New Bridge and the Blackfriars Settlement.

A Conflict of Traditions?

When, after approximately a century of parallel existence, probation and after-care were unified in 1965 (in response to the ACTO Report) there was a conflict of tradition. Probation could claim by then to be professional. Links with its voluntary roots had become tenuous. But after-care represented an unbroken tradition of voluntary service.

Not surprisingly probation officers were apprehensive about reintroducing volunteers. The arguments for doing so in the ACTO Report[14] did not seem persuasive. Why, when the report seemed so critical of the discharged prisoners' aid societies, should the new Probation and After-Care Service be expected to make room for their voluntary workers? Faced with the problem of devising effective help for a more damaged and hardened group of clients, how convincing was the argument that the 'main need of many offenders is for simple encouragement, friendship and human understanding'? Did the statement that the Probation and After-Care Service would be unable to undertake the formidable new duties unaided imply that adequate professional staff would not be forthcoming—a recipe for undermining professional standards? In brief was the object of the merger to raise the standards of after-care to that of probation or to dilute probation with an influx of sub-professional workers?

Given time, some probation officers began to see not a conflict of traditions, but a marriage of the new professionalism with a rediscovered voluntary tradition. Volunteers were in any case playing a bigger part in other social services and social work theory had become much broader with growing emphasis upon the community and utilizing its resources. But in the short run much damage was done. Few of the previous voluntary associates linked up with the new Probation and After-Care Service, and many of the voluntary supporters of the discharged prisoners' aid societies were lost (although some of the societies rechannelled their efforts into providing after-care hostels).

A Belated Response

However, a marked increase in the number of volunteers recruited in 1967–8 by the Probation and After-Care Service can be seen as a belated response to the ACTO Report, reinforced by Home Office encouragement[15] and the second report[16] of Lady Reading's Working Party.

A survey of probation and after-care services in England and Wales for the period up to 31 December 1966 showed that only thirty-five were involving volunteers. A similar survey giving the position on 31 December 1968 found that 48 were doing so.* During the intervening two years 1,204 volunteers (582 men and 622 women) had been recruited in addition to the 794 recruited previously (of whom some would have withdrawn).

During the last quarter of 1968, 1,223 volunteers had been used although no breakdown of the information is available to show how many were involved, respectively, as voluntary associates giving long-term help to offenders, as volunteers working with offenders' families, or as volunteers undertaking short-term practical tasks. Indeed, many were probably involved in a combination of two or all of these, making a detailed analysis difficult. The figures do, however, give two pointers regarding the 'voluntary associate' type of work. Whereas in 1966 only 3 areas had had volunteers visiting offenders during sentence, by 1968 the number had risen to 40 and 326 volunteers were doing so. While this implies a sharp increase it also reveals that the large majority of volunteers were still solely involved with the offender after discharge or with his family.

Figures extracted from Probation Statistics for 1966 and 1967 show that the number of persons 'befriended' on release rose from 18,522 to 22,441. In 1966 volunteers were involved in 444 of these cases and in 1967 in 1,075 of them, an increase from 2·4 per cent to 4·8 per cent.

Although it remains a very small proportion of the after-care cases, there is a marked increase. These figures do not, of course, mean that volunteers were involved in helping 4·8 per cent of all men and women released, as the majority of them did not come to the Probation and After-

---

* In 1966 there were 84 probation and after-care committees of whom 83 replied. In 1968 there were 82 committees of whom 77 replied. The remaining 5 were all in rural areas and 2 of them only employed part-time staff.

Care Service for help, or if they did so, came only on an occasional and casual basis.

Vercoe[17] in a report of the National Association for the Care and Resettlement of Offenders (NACRO) described the work of volunteers with prisoners' families. During 1967 she visited 43 probation and after-care areas which had been randomly selected and found that in 29 areas using volunteers, just under three-quarters made use of them for long-term contact with families. In the remaining areas they were used to visit for a specific purpose, or to perform practical tasks such as transporting furniture. The report also found that in two-thirds of the areas visited use was made of voluntary organizations to help prisoners' families. The only one on a national scale was WRVS and half the officers using it did so purely for practical tasks.

Different Pattern of Development
The pattern of development has differed from area to area, and obviously the need for volunteers varies. In rural areas, for example, the number of ex-prisoners returning is much smaller than in large cities or industrial conurbations. In addition, it may be possible to draw upon existing sources of community support more easily in rural areas as and when these are needed, without the setting up of organized voluntary services. At the other extreme, in London the scale and nature of the problem was much greater and necessitated a totally different approach in which existing voluntary organizations were invited to play a major part. The development of a uniform practice by probation and after-care committees would have been inappropriate, ignoring the local situation, and restricting the scope for experimentation.

But voluntary associate schemes have not been exclusively in the major centres of population. One of the first, following the ACTO Report, was started by Pendleton[18] in Rugby in March 1964, with fourteen 'voluntary helpers' and is important for the stress put upon training and supervision.

Several other new projects linked with the probation services have been described in short articles and give some idea of developments in provincial cities: Thompson[19] (Oxford), Worthy[20] (Birmingham), and Baillie[21] (Birkenhead).

Lingering Doubts among the Professionals
But despite the growing number of volunteers many probation officers still tended to see them as a means of coping with short-term practical

jobs—collecting luggage, arranging transport for a wife to visit her husband in prison, or baby-sitting. There was reluctance to accept the idea of a voluntary associate who might have a long-term and personal relationship with a client. The gradual acceptance of this role for the voluntary associate would alter the contribution of the probation officer himself. As Miles[22] noted, the probation officer 'will no longer be able to work with every case by the formation and use of a relationship. . . . His role in many instances will be to provide the support and guidance to the auxiliaries [volunteers] who will develop their own relationship with the client.'

Many probation officers were still sceptical about the reliability of voluntary associates and were naturally apprehensive about handing over their cases to them. They were, however, more willing to do so if the voluntary associate was known to them personally and they could have some say in his selection for the particular client. Similarly, they had more confidence in voluntary associates who they, or their colleagues, had helped to train and select.

Individual Volunteers without Voluntary Organizations

It followed from this that the most acceptable way of recruiting voluntary associates was as individuals to work directly under the auspices of the Probation and After-Care Service, thus enabling the probation officer to supervise their work and to retain overall responsibility for the clients. As a result, voluntary organizations which in the past had had clients referred to them by probation officers for long-term supportive help found that their source of supply was drying up.

It would be misleading to imply that the voluntary organizations were totally squeezed out of such work, but the number of referrals fell sharply and their role became limited in most areas to practical short-term jobs rather than long-term involvement with clients or their families. This exclusion in most areas of the voluntary organization from voluntary associate work was reinforced by the recommendations of the second Reading Report.[23]

Voluntary Associates

But it is with such work that this report is concerned. Since 1922 there had been prison visitors, another group of volunteers, regularly interviewing prisoners, in their cells, but with little or no contact after discharge, indeed it had been discouraged. The voluntary associates introduced after the Maxwell Report shifted the emphasis to after-care, so that the pre-discharge contact was seen as preliminary. The voluntary associates' allegiance was to the outside after-care society rather than to the prison. Thus two kinds of volunteer coexisted.

Teamwork Associates and other projects introduced after the 1965 reorganization of after-care were a means by which the new Probation and After-Care Service could gain experience of involving voluntary associates. They also helped the service to crystallize some of its thinking about its new after-care duties and about the relationship between the professional and the volunteer.

REFERENCES

1. John Kent, *Elizabeth Fry*, Batsford 1962, and other biographies.
2. C. Leeson (ed.), *The Probation System*, P. S. King & Son 1914.
3. The Report of the Departmental Committee on the Training, Appointment and Payment of Probation Officers, HMSO 1922.
4. L. Le Mesurier (ed.), *A Handbook of Probation*, National Association of Probation Officers 1935, p. 70.
5. The Report of the Departmental Committee on the Social Services in the Courts of Summary Jurisdiction, HMSO 1936.
6. Gordon Hamilton, *Theory and Practice of Social Casework*, Columbia University Press 1940, p. 22.
7. Helen Harris Perlman, *Social Casework: A Problem Solving Process*, University of Chicago Press 1957, p. 65.
8. Felix Biestek, *The Casework Relationship*, George Allen and Unwin 1961. First published in the USA 1957.
9. See Probation Research Project, Steven Folkard and others, *A Preliminary Report*, A Home Office Research Unit Report, HMSO 1966, Table 16.
10. The Report of the Departmental Committee on the Probation Service, HMSO, 1962, par. 59.
11. Op. cit.
12. The Report of the Committee on Discharged Prisoners' Aid Societies, HMSO, 1953, Ch. 4.
13. A. W. Lacey, *The Role of Voluntary Effort in the After-Care of Offenders*, unpublished Ph.D. thesis, London School of Economics 1963. See Also A. W. Lacey, 'The Citizen and After-Care', *The Howard Journal*, Vol. XI No. 3 1964.
14. Op. cit., p. 35.
15. Home Office Circular 238/1965. (See Appendix to the Second Reading Report.)
16. Op. cit.
17. Kate Vercoe, *Helping Prisoners' Families*, Papers and Reprints No. 3, NACRO 1968, p. 10.

18. John Pendleton, *The Rugby Scheme for Voluntary Helpers in After-Care*, Appendix 1 in *Casework in After-Care*, Mark Monger, Butterworth 1967.

19. K. D. Thompson, *Voluntary Social Workers: An Oxford Experiment*, Probation Vol. 11 No. 1, March 1965.

20. A. Worthy, *Voluntary After-Care Workers*, Justice of the Peace and Local Government Review, 22 February 1969.

21. David Baillie, *Charlie Come Home*, Probation Vol. 13 No. 2.

22. Ieuan Miles, *Probation and After-Care*, Probation Papers No. 3, National Association of Probation Officers 1966.

23. Op. cit., pars 22–3.

CHAPTER 2

THE PROJECT

The Presenting Problem
Almost invariably initiative in voluntary action springs from direct en-
counter with people in need and this project was no exception. In
April 1964, a working party of twelve Christian Teamwork* members
was convened 'to investigate the problems of finding work for ex-
prisoners' following several requests to that organization to help ex-
prisoners with employment problems.

Although work was not infrequently a difficulty it soon became clear
to the working party that it could not be dealt with in isolation from the
ex-prisoner's total needs. According to the Pakenham-Thompson Committee[1] the problem for many ex-prisoners lay not in finding but in
keeping employment. This suggested that their problems were related
to their ability to maintain acceptable relationships in the outside world.

Defining the Task
This trend of thought prompted a broader enquiry into the responsibility
of the community in general, and the churches in particular, towards
the ex-prisoner. The working party noted the proposals in the then
recently published ACTO Report[2] to stimulate renewed effort by voluntary workers and, in particular, the importance attached to the churches
as a source of support.

Initially a proposal was drafted for a pilot project in London to
mobilize the active participation of the churches in after-care, but the

* Christian Teamwork, established in 1957, is an interdenominational organization which provided a consultative service seeking to give help which combined
professional competence with Christian understanding. It was to this service that
several prison welfare officers turned for help in finding work for men on discharge.
In 1966 the Christian Teamwork Trust set up a separate Institute, now called the
Grubb Institute of Behavioural Studies, to make more widely known the results of
its earlier work, and to provide opportunities to learn about human behaviour
through education and research.

working party soon came to see that to set up an exclusively Christian organization might divide the resources of the community in an unhelpful way.

As a result, the aims of the project were broadened to explore means of mobilizing the resources of the community to help in the resettlement of ex-prisoners. Within this broad aim it was hoped to give special attention to the role of the churches and Christian organizations. More specifically the aims of the project were defined as follows:

1. To recruit, train, select, and ensure professional support for voluntary associates.
2. To provide voluntary associates to befriend prisoners during and after sentence, primarily in Inner London.*
3. To evaluate systematically the development of the project during an initial period of three years and to publish a report on it.

After much debate it was decided to adopt the name 'Teamwork Associates' to link the name of the founding organization Christian Teamwork with the phrase 'voluntary associates'. The word 'teamwork' was also an apt description of the intention to organize the work into local teams and to encourage partnership between professionals and volunteers.

A Beginning

During these vital planning stages there were many setbacks, not least the uncertainty as to how far the proposals were welcome to the statutory authorities. The preference of most probation and after-care committees for the direct recruitment of voluntary associates[3] did not encourage confidence in the future of a new voluntary organization. However, the Inner London Probation and After-Care Committee expressed confidence in the potential value of the project and urged the working party to proceed. Encouraged by this, it saw the opportunity to develop a project with a voluntary identity yet working in the closest co-operation with the statutory services.

Thus on 5 May 1966 the inaugural meeting was held to establish

* The Inner London Probation and After-Care Area comprises the twelve inner boroughs, approximately, covering the same area as the former London County Council. It has a population of approximately 3¼ million with individual boroughs varying between 204,000 and 340,000. Outer London was the responsibility of four separate probation and after-care committees which were not involved with the project. (Figures as for 1 April 1965.)

Teamwork Associates as a company limited by guarantee, and it was subsequently registered as a charity and accredited by the Inner London Probation and After-Care Committee.

The working party was augmented to become the project committee and a number of distinguished persons with known sympathies for the work lent their names as sponsors.

On the 1 June the writer took up the position of director, having been appointed on secondment as a probation officer by the Inner London Probation and After-Care Committee.

Gaining Recognition

In the early stages there were difficulties in gaining recognition from the community, from the Probation and After-Care Service and from other voluntary after-care organizations.

It soon became clear that 'Teamwork Associates', although an apt name in the opinion of the insiders, had no obvious meaning to outsiders. In a field of work crowded with small voluntary organizations, some of which were well known, it was difficult to obtain recognition. Too much publicity might have the effect of offending other organizations in the same field with whom the project would need to work closely.

Opinion in the Probation and After-Care Service was against advertising for voluntary associates and was wary about the effects of press comments or articles in magazines. It was feared that such publicity would attract a large proportion of unsuitable voluntary associates. While there was little evidence to support these fears, Teamwork Associates was disinclined to take the risk by embarking upon a publicity campaign.

The Participation of Other Organizations

It had, in any case, been decided to concentrate on appeals to existing bodies inviting them to provide members to do the work within the framework of their own organization, rather than to set out to attract individuals direct. In the first instance, it was hoped to enlist support within the churches.

The process of gaining the active participation of organizations inevitably took longer than a direct appeal by advertising for individuals. This, plus a disappointing response from most, though not all, of the churches, resulted in very slow recruitment during the early months. Often there was a time lag, contacts made in the first few months prompting support much later. Even when the response was more immediate there was still a period of five or six months between the initial recruitment of individuals from the organizations and the subsequent accreditation of the voluntary associate after a preparation course.

Pressure of Numbers
The effect of this slow start was to prompt pressure from the Probation and After-Care Service, and others, to accelerate the rate of recruitment. Only by increasing the rate of growth, it seemed, would the project be taken seriously by the Probation and After-Care Service and, incidentally, be accepted by other voluntary after-care organizations as a going concern.

To yield to these pressures, it was realized, might prevent the director from giving sufficient time to recording, planning and evaluating, which were the essence of a pilot project. There was the temptation to embark on ambitious, large-scale plans without first establishing the need for, or effectiveness of, the service offered. After much discussion it was agreed to accelerate development, but to resist any invitation to extend beyond Inner London or beyond the boundaries of voluntary associate work with individual offenders, at least until the three years were completed. As a result the director was still able to give some time to reflection on progress, although the evaluation of the project was less intensive and less systematic than it might have been. On the other hand, many questions of organization and co-operation with the Probation and After-Care Service had to be tackled, which would not have been the case had the project consisted, throughout, of a handful of voluntary associates working exclusively with the director.

There was, however, another major effect of the decision to expand. It was clear from the disappointing response of the churches, that the project could not rely heavily upon them as a source of recruits. Only by exploring all possible methods of recruitment, including contacts with many other organizations and more publicity, could numbers be increased.

But many of those who volunteered to help subsequently were motivated by religious belief and, in this, the project reflected a long-standing tradition in voluntary service. However, the link with the institutional church did not develop as strongly as had been hoped. In its place, close partnership was established with several voluntary organizations, especially councils of social service, but the most significant change was in the increased recruitment of individuals thus departing to some extent from the original emphasis upon working through organizations.

The End of the First Year
By the end of the first year most of these teething troubles had been resolved. After about nine months the flow of volunteers began to increase and from then on remained fairly steady. At the same time the earlier volunteers were beginning to reach the stage of accreditation and to make contact with their first clients. By the end of the year twenty-nine had become accredited voluntary associates.

Decentralization
For the first nine months the director had acted as consultant to all the voluntary associates in two teams, one based at his office in the After-Care Registry and Resettlement Unit and the other at a central church. As numbers increased it was decided to divide the voluntary associates into smaller teams to be located in various boroughs of Inner London and to work closely with the local probation officers, from whom they would take referrals and have support. Six teams were started initially.

This decentralization marked a vital point in the development of the project and its partnership with the Probation and After-Care Service. It was the first time that a voluntary after-care organization had placed its members with the statutory service, thus relinquishing much of its own control. This involved some risk. Would relations between probation officers and voluntary associates deteriorate, or would they work towards a realistic and positive partnership?

Borough Teams
Each of these teams, and those set up later, developed its own character. Only one disintegrated and that was later restarted with the help of the same senior probation officer. Much of the credit for getting them started must go to the probation officers who were invited to act as 'consultants' to the teams. Despite their inexperience in the use of voluntary associates, they were willing to accept a great deal of dependence from them and to undertake this additional and demanding work. In all, over 20 probation officers acted as consultants.

Borough Projects
Some teams had roots in their local community but others had not, although the voluntary associates lived within reasonable travelling distance. In making plans to start teams in other boroughs it was decided to contact organization which might act as 'recruiting agents' within

the area. It was in the Borough of Camden that the first opportunity arose to attempt a large scale 'recruiting campaign' at borough level and a departure from the original reluctance to advertise. A partnership with the Camden Council of Social Service was established and its staff contributed knowledge of their borough, professional skill in the mobil-ization of community support and, by no means least, enthusiasm. The experience in Camden set a pattern for the future.

In the Borough of Lewisham, the promising start made in Camden was repeated with the Lewisham Council of Social Service, again with encouraging results. This reinforced the director's conviction that the project had now hit upon an effective method to provoke community interest and action. Not all Inner London Boroughs have their own councils of social service so it was not possible to repeat the experience everywhere. Nor would it have been reasonable to expect them all to allocate such a substantial part of their energies to prison after-care, but the response both in the boroughs and by the London Council of Social Service who publicized the project,[4] was most encouraging. It indicated a willingness by those in the mainstream of voluntary social service to see the needs of offenders as part of their responsibility rather than as an isolated problem to be dealt with solely by specialist agen-cies.

In the Borough of Wandsworth local publicity was again used and International Voluntary Services helped to recruit members for a local team. Shortly after the end of the second year teams had been started in 10 of the 12 Inner London Boroughs. Appendix Table A shows the distribution of the voluntary associates in the various boroughs.

Local Courses

The increasing tempo of the project could be sustained only by running more preparation courses and basing them in the boroughs where local recruitment was initiated. From the Spring of 1967 two courses were run each term. Often each was locally based in a borough where recruiting was in progress, but some were held centrally to cater for individuals from other boroughs and to top up the numbers in teams already estab-lished.

This scale of activity could not have been maintained without the enthusiastic support of probation officers as co-tutors with the director, and as speakers. Again they started without any previous experience, but learned perhaps as much from the courses as did the members.

Levelling Out

At the end of the second year a total of 94 voluntary associates had been accepted, of whom 8 had subsequently withdrawn. The preoccupation of the director, up to this point, had been with recruitment, training and selection. It was now necessary to switch the emphasis by reducing the rate of recruitment and working much more closely with the consultant probation officers who were beginning to involve the growing number of voluntary associates in the work.

Consultants' Group

To facilitate exchange of experience between different teams and to enable the director (who no longer had a team himself) to have some involvement in the field work, the consultants agreed to meet every second month.

Conferences and Social Occasions

Similarly opportunities were provided for the voluntary associates to meet centrally every 4 to 6 months either for a conference to discuss the progress of the project or some aspect of the work, or for a social occasion. These gatherings, which were well attended and greatly appreciated, were initiated principally as a means of retaining a corporate identity for the scattered teams.

The Development of the Teams

Some teams gained in confidence and morale more quickly than others. Some retained a strong sense of identity with Teamwork Associates, while one or two identified much more with the Probation and After-Care Service locally. Early in the third year it began to look as if the localized organization with the close links with the probation officers would fragment Teamwork Associates into a series of separate groups, each of which might become increasingly identified with the statutory service. But most of the voluntary associates and the consultants, since then, have indicated their need for a cohesive voluntary identity.

In several respects the development of the teams differed little. All had difficulty in obtaining enough referrals from probation officers in the first three months or so, and sometimes for longer. In most instances the referrals by the consultant from his own caseload, supported by those from one or two of his colleagues, produced enough clients, but the problem of balancing supply and demand was always difficult.

In most teams, initial dependence upon the consultant gradually eased, with signs of wanting a measure of separation from the probation officers, but in only two teams did the members appoint their own conveners. In the remainder the probation officer acted as both convener and consultant, although he often enlisted the help of a voluntary associate as honorary secretary.

Effects of Decentralization on the Type of Client
The decentralization of the voluntary associates to the boroughs left the After-Care Registry and Resettlement Unit as the base for the project, but not so fully involved as during the first few months. It was this Unit which catered for the homeless ex-prisoner, a type of client thought, at first, to be in special need of a link with the community, perhaps through a voluntary associate. However, experience showed that many of the clients dealt with by the Unit were psychologically far too damaged, too drifting and too unable to form relationships to be helped by a voluntary associate, although there were exceptions. The majority saw their needs solely in terms of aid on discharge and came to the Unit as 'casual callers'. Working, instead, with the probation officers in the boroughs, the voluntary associates were more likely to be in touch with prisoners or ex-prisoners with a settled address but many were still of a lonely and rootless disposition. Devolution to the boroughs also led to requests to help prisoners' families, probationers and other clients who had not been in institutions.

Homeless Young Offenders
In April 1968 the Inner London Probation and After-Care Service took over responsibility from the former Borstal After-Care Association for all borstal after-care in Inner London. It was decided that those young men who were expected to be homeless on discharge would be the responsibility of a group of probation officers at the After-Care Registry and Resettlement Unit and the scheme for liaison probation officers to prisons would be extended to borstals so that contact could be made early in the sentence.

The chronic instability and high reconviction rates of homeless young men discharged from borstal was fully recognized, as was the need for an imaginative approach to mobilize all available sources of help. To this end the Inner London Probation and After-Care Service invited Teamwork Associates to join it in sponsoring a 'Youth Resettlement Project', to mobilize the resources of the community through individuals and organizations to provide support and practical help for homeless young people returning to Inner London on discharge from borstal institutions. Initially it was to be for young men from borstal, but later to include girls, and those who had been 'young prisoners' or were licensed from detention centres. Two probation officers were assigned as project officers, each to give half his time to the project, and the other half mainly to borstal after-care duties within the Unit. It is hoped to publish a report on the project later.

The Shepton Mallet Project

Another development, but on a smaller scale, was started by the borough team in Kensington which established a small group of voluntary associates to visit long-term inmates regularly at Shepton Mallet Prison, Somerset some 180 miles away. Many of these men were likely to be homeless on discharge and posed special problems, both in and out of the institution, because of the types of sex offences for which many of them had been convicted. The project was designed to provide an informal group meeting in the prison in which voluntary associates and prisoners could establish a relationship.

After Three Years

At the end of the project 155 accredited voluntary associates were actively involved with Teamwork Associates, in 10 borough teams and a further 4 teams comprising the Youth Resettlement Project. Although the rate of growth in the boroughs had been steadied during the final year, the promising start of the Youth Resettlement Project compensated for this, sustaining the overall rate of growth.

In the following chapters we shall be considering in more detail some of the subjects touched upon in this general description of the project.

REFERENCES

1. *Problems of the Ex-prisoner*, A Report of the Pakenham-Thompson Committee, pp. 13–14, National Council of Social Service 1961.
   See also J. P. Martin, *Offenders as Employees*, Cambridge Studies in Criminology, 1962.
2. Op. cit., pars 120–2, 128.
3. Op. cit., pars 9–10, 21.
4. *Opportunities for Voluntary Service*, London Council of Social Service, revised and reprinted regularly.

CHAPTER 3

RECRUITMENT

The lifeblood of the project, as the previous chapter illustrated, was the recruitment of a sufficient number of able and committed voluntary associates. The ACTO Report[1] was assured by its witnesses 'that many people would come forward to offer voluntary service as auxiliaries if a call were made to them in terms both clear and practical telling them how and where their help was required'. The report gave the following as some 'likely recruiting grounds': local prisoners' aid societies, existing voluntary associate schemes, prison visitors, the churches, 'various national voluntary organizations', and many persons unattached to any voluntary organization.

The subsequent Home Office Circular[2] stressed the practical advantages of recruiting volunteers through community organizations. It was this advice which Teamwork Associates sought to follow in the early stages of the project.

The Churches
As reported in the previous chapter, much time was given during the first year of the project to trying to enlist support from local churches. In all, 92 were approached during the year, these being chosen on the advice of members of the Committee who through, for example, the British Council of Churches or Christian Teamwork were well informed regarding churches with a lively interest in social problems. Letters were sent to clergy, enclosing an outline of the project, and an offer by the director to visit. Despite the temptation to assign yet another request for help to the wastepaper bin, nearly half the clergy invited the director to call and most of them expressed interest. Requests to write short articles for church magazines and to speak to mid-week meetings were accepted in many instances. Contact was established also with central bodies concerned with citizenship or social responsibility by the churches, again with encouraging signs of interest and some publicity through the religious press.

In view of the good will shown, the failure to obtain practical offers of help from more than two or three churches was the more disappointing. In two boroughs, local churches recruited members for courses. Numbers at the beginning were large, but the rate of drop-out during the courses was also large, perhaps as a result of some press-gang tactics in the first place. Of those who completed the courses and applied to become voluntary associates, again a larger than average proportion was rejected, confirming the impression gained by tutors during the courses regarding the calibre of some members. As a result it was impossible to set up church-based groups as had been hoped.

The Councils of Social Service

The ability of the Councils of Social Service in some areas to become key recruiting agents for voluntary associates, as noted in the previous chapter, was just one example of their role in stimulating the participation of volunteers throughout the health and social services. The setting up of a 'Voluntary Workers' Bureau', especially if it has full-time professional staff as in Camden, provides a channel through which potential volunteers, many of whom have no strong preference for one particular field of service can find a niche which fits their interests, aptitudes and available time.

Such bureaux are growing in number and the Aves Report recommended their extension.[3] The experience of the project suggests that they could take a major responsibility in the recruitment of voluntary associates, providing their staff were properly briefed so that they were aware of the qualities required, and skilled in conducting some initial screening (without being made responsible for subsequent selection).

Other Voluntary Organizations

Approaches to other voluntary organizations during the project tended to be piecemeal and it would be misleading to draw firm conclusions. At various times approaches were made to Toc H, Rotary, Settlements, Trade Unions, Trades Councils and organizations of young volunteers, such as International Voluntary Service (IVS), Task Force, Volunteers Overseas Service Association (VOSA) and student groups.

A few Toc H members attended courses as did several members of Rotary, although the latter seemed better suited to offer professional or business skills of the kind needed, for example, in a hostel project. The Settlements were already actively involved through the Blackfriars Scheme and the Hammersmith Voluntary After-Care Scheme, but

Toynbee Hall found a number of voluntary associates and became the base for the Tower Hamlets team, while Cambridge House through its Literacy Scheme found voluntary associates for the Youth Resettlement Project.

Although several contacts were made with senior members of the Trade Union Movement and with one Trades Council early in the project, there was little response. It would be unfair to assume that more help could not have been found with a greater effort and more understanding about the Movement, although efforts in other areas seem to have been equally unsuccessful.

The role of organizations for young volunteers was clearly limited in a field of work where it was generally agreed that an older and more mature person was needed. But there was the possibility of attracting the 'not-so-young volunteer', who had perhaps tired of the work-camp type of activities or found them incompatible with family responsibilities. On this basis several members of IVS were recruited.

The Youth Resettlement Project has actively explored recruitment through the young volunteer organizations, but it has not proved possible to involve students while still at university or college because the long-term nature of voluntary associate work conflicts with short academic terms and the need to break off voluntary service at examination times.

By Probation Officers and Prison Staff

In some areas outside London recruitment seems to have been done by personal invitation from probation officers. Where there is only a limited need for voluntary associates this may be an adequate means of finding them and ensures that the individuals concerned are acceptable to the probation officers.

In Inner London, Teamwork Associates found that one or two probation officers were alert to the possibility of recruitment when meeting helpful members of the public in the course of their daily work. Similarly, one prison governor and his welfare officers, forwarded names of those who had written in offering help. Given the same alertness throughout the Probation and After-Care Service and at the local prisons, there can be little doubt that many potential voluntary associates would be found. There might also be many among those who approach the Home Office or principal probation officers about becoming probation officers but either do not apply or are turned down on educational grounds.

By other Voluntary Associates

Only a few voluntary associates were recruited by other voluntary associates, which may seem surprising. One explanation would seem to be that they wanted to find their feet in the job and to make sure that it was feasible before involving their friends. Another difficulty may have been the fear that in the event of their friends being rejected or running into serious difficulties in the work, their own relationship with them might have been strained.

Talks, Radio and Television

Most talks about the project were given to churches and organizations mentioned above. The response in offers of help was minimal, but the talks may be seen as part of the slow process of influencing public opinion and creating, in the most general sense, a less prejudiced and more accepting response to the ex-offender.

Like these talks, participation in radio and television programmes was more likely to have an indirect than a direct effect, upon the recruitment of voluntary associates. Often the programme had only an oblique relevance to voluntary associate work, and covered a much wider area than that in which recruits were being sought.

Articles, Press Comments and Advertisements

Most articles written during the project to attract voluntary associates were for magazines or journals with a small circulation and again, often tied in with attempts to involve members of a particular organization. Content tended to be factual with only a restrained use of disguised case studies, for fear of stimulating a flood of replies triggered off by an emotional appeal.

From time to time such articles prompted reports in local newspapers, or enquiries from journalists which were not discouraged, although no attempt was made to report on the project 'in depth'.

To pep up the rate of recruitment when necessary, or to stimulate developments in particular boroughs, simple advertisements were inserted in newspapers and journals inviting enrolment for a course 'to learn about how to help ex-prisoners'. Local evening newspapers and the religious weeklies produced little response, but the *New Statesman* could be relied upon to produce results although not necessarily in the local areas. Not surprisingly these enquirers tended to be drawn from left-wing intellectual backgrounds.

Leaflets

Simple leaflets were also prepared for distribution to interested individuals. One of these, entitled 'The Second Sentence ?' argued that the
prisoner's real punishment began not on the day of sentence but on the
day of discharge and appealed for him to be given a fair chance. 'If you
believe', it read, 'that an ex-prisoner has paid his debt, please consider
what you could do. . . .' Other leaflets simply set out a programme for
the next course and in a few words explained its purpose. All but one of
these were in duplicated form and to do without good quality printed
literature was probably a false economy.

Dangers of Publicity

Despite earlier apprehension about publicity its use did not produce any
obvious increase in the number of enquirers who were unsuitable, using
a non-emotive theme and advertising the preparation course rather than
the job itself. All the above methods of recruitment, not just publicity,
produced a proportion of enquirers who were clearly unsuitable and the
initial interview and screening process had to be geared to detecting
them and, if possible, dissuading them at the outset.

The Rate of Recruitment

Although no one method of recruitment, with the possible exception of
Councils of Social Service, was strikingly successful, the overall response
was sufficient to meet the needs of a pilot project. The main regulating
factors were the number of places available on courses and the gradual
development of a feeling in the Probation and After-Care Service that
more voluntary associates would be needed. To have increased numbers
faster than the demand for their service would have invited disillusion.

Social Class

Whether the voluntary associates were being found from the right social
class was a matter of opinion. As Chapter 7 shows, they were predominantly middle-class. The second Reading Report[4] called for effort
and imagination to break away from this traditional source of volunteers,
and the same sentiment has often been repeated since. In practice, this
is a far from simple issue and one which we shall consider later (p. 131).

How the Voluntary Associates Came

In the light of the above discussion it may be of interest to note how the

121 voluntary associates who completed the questionnaire said that they first heard of the project. Their answers are given in Table 1.

TABLE 1

How the Voluntary Associates First Heard About the Work

	%
Advertisements, articles, TV or radio	20·6
Church or Christian organizations	19·8
Personal contacts of voluntary associates and project supporters	17·3
Probation officers	15·8
Councils of social service	12·4
Other	14·1
N = 121	100·0

Care must be taken in drawing deductions from these figures. For example, many of those listed as responding to advertisements or press comments were part of 'recruiting campaigns' launched with councils of social service. Thus the figure recruited with their help was more than the 12·4 per cent stated. Any comparison between the number recruited through, for example, churches as against councils of social service must take account of the fact that there were over a hundred of the former and primarily two of the latter. However, the figures are included to give a general picture of the sources of recruitment.

REFERENCES

1. Op. cit., pars 125–30.
2. Op. cit., pars 13–14.
3. Op. cit., par. 296.
4. Op. cit., par. 35.

CHAPTER 4

MOTIVATION

By one or other of the methods described in the previous chapter, many thousands of people received the invitation to offer their help, yet the number actually volunteering can be counted in hundreds. The experience confirms the belief that the vast majority of the public do not want to know about the needs of the ex-prisoner, or see him as a 'problem' to be coped with by the official services—police, prison, probation and so on. Even for those who were predisposed to give voluntary service the more 'deserving' claims of the young, the aged and the handicapped, had perhaps a more positive emotional appeal.

What then prompted a member of the public to step out of line, sometimes in the face of criticism from family or friends, by volunteering to help ex-prisoners? In some fields of voluntary service to ask questions about applicants' motivation is regarded as unnecessary or even improper. It is considered enough that they should want to help. But in a field such as after-care, where motives may affect attitudes to the work and relationships with clients constructively or destructively, it is a question which calls for detailed investigation in some depth. The following comments arise simply from several hundred interviews with enquirers and from discussions during courses for voluntary associates.

That people should try to help without payment and in their own time sometimes prompted a client to question their motives. Similarly probation officers have wondered to what extent voluntary associates were seeking to satisfy their own needs, and maybe to resolve their own problems, by doing voluntary work, though the same can be true of professional workers.

The motives, conscious and unconscious, which prompt an offer of service are complex and subtle. Any attempt to isolate particular factors for the purpose of discussion involves over-simplification. Perhaps the only generalization that can be made safely is that every voluntary associate is motivated by a mixture of altruism and self-interest. The measure of his recognition of the latter may be an indication of his awareness and his ability to see the relationship with the client as reciprocal, each party finding some fulfilment of his needs. Such a relationship is likely to be free from the taint of patronage which results when one party sees himself as purely altruistic, acting only to satisfy the needs of the other.

In Place of Professional Social Work

One motivating factor seemed to be a desire to gain experience before applying for professional social work training. Similarly voluntary associate work sometimes seems to be a compensation for not being able to make an application, or being unsuccessful in doing so.

The first of these factors was more common among young people not settled in their career or married women contemplating paid employment when the children grew up. These felt that voluntary associate work would offer a greater degree of involvement with clients than most other types of voluntary work and the chance to gain useful experience with initial preparation and ongoing professional support. Perhaps more important for some was the opportunity to test themselves against the demands of a difficult form of work before deciding whether to expose themselves to similar pressures on a full-time basis. Many social studies and social work courses expect their students to have had some relevant experience before accepting them and being a voluntary associate may be regarded as such.

As the opportunities for voluntary service increase, so a larger proportion of students are likely to have some experience of it. This has considerable advantages. Some of the trials of students during and immediately after professional training may be eased. Particularly important in the present context, they may retain in their subsequent career a lively awareness of the volunteer, based upon first-hand experience. On the other hand, while volunteers themselves, they are likely to differ from their fellows. Experience during the project suggested that those for whom social work aspirations were a motivating factor identified more closely with the professional workers than did other voluntary associates. There was a risk that they would want to extend their understanding and their learning beyond the boundaries of the voluntary associates' role, by trying to adopt the professionals' attitudes and skills in anticipation of their professional careers. These were hazards to be watched, and to be discussed with those concerned, though they seemed less worrying as the scope of the voluntary associates' contribution gradually broadened.

Those for whom frustration in failing to enter professional social work was a factor were usually older. Some had applied too late in life to be considered for training; some lacked the requisite educational qualifications; others had not applied because of family responsibilities or because it would have resulted in a drop in income which they could not have afforded.

Religious Beliefs

We have already noted the origins of voluntary associate work in the Christian traditions of the last century. Although the church as an institution did not find as many voluntary associates for the project as had been hoped, a factor which frequently seemed to prompt individual offers of help was the concern to give practical expression to Christian beliefs. Those for whom this seemed to be a motivating factor represented a diverse cross-section of denominational groups and ranged from those who were deeply involved in the life of their local church to those whose links were more tenuous. Many of them saw becoming a voluntary associate as a way of helping people with whom they would be unlikely to make contact in the course of their church activities. In this sense they could claim to be the modern missionaries, but with the noticeable absence of moralizing or misplaced evangelism.

Amongst the enquirers there were, however, those whose primary concern was the conversion of the ex-prisoner, and who found it difficult to see how a Christian could help if this was not central. During the preparation courses and the selection procedure, this was often discussed, stressing the right of the client to live his own life, and the danger of abusing a privileged relationship in which the client was at some disadvantage. Most evangelical Christians either readily accepted this point of view or were prepared to go along with it, but there were a few who declined to apply to become voluntary associates within an organization which seemed too restrictive. This did not result in the loss of all those of evangelical tradition, many of whom contributed greatly to the project, as they have in the professional social work field; nor did it deny the Christian the right to speak openly of his faith to his client providing this was encouraged, and just so long as it was encouraged, by the latter.

In addition to those prompted by Christian conviction, there were those similarly motivated by their Jewish faith, again reflecting a long-standing tradition of social service.

Political Beliefs

A further factor was political beliefs, usually of a left-wing intellectual kind, and these seemed to be associated with an interest in penal reform, as well as in helping the individual offender. However, the voluntary associates concerned did not seem to experience any great difficulty in working within a penal system which they wished to see changed, without feeling that they were giving tacit approval to all its practices.

There was much to be said for including in the project some who were inclined to look critically at authority and established practices, providing this did not interfere with its practical work for clients. At an early stage it was feared that political motives would be linked with a tendency to collude with the client against authority as represented by the probation officer, but in practice this did not become a problem.

Personal Needs

Some voluntary associates felt the need to help to repay for their good fortune in life, but this seemed to spring from a sense of moral obligation rather than guilt about the inequalities of life.

Others felt a need to compensate for a lack of fulfilment in their daily work, frequently because there was little scope for personal involvement with people, or for a similar deficiency in their interests or family life. Sometimes they, too, were lonely or found it difficult to find acceptance in the community, and here there was a risk of exploiting the client to meet the voluntary associate's need. On the other hand, the experience of successfully surmounting a personal problem, or learning to live with it, seemed to enhance the capacity of some voluntary associates to understand and to identify with the client in his problems.

Direct Experience of Ex-prisoners

A few voluntary associates were interested initially by meeting an ex-prisoner, or knowing someone who had fallen foul of the law and had been imprisoned. Experience of trying to help one individual had sometimes led to a concern to help others and to an awareness of the need for some preparation and links with the Probation and After-Care Service for support.

Reasons given by Voluntary Associates

When a person applied to become a voluntary associate he was asked to record on his application his reason for wishing to take up the work. Many found this difficult and some answers like 'to help ex-prisoners' were reasonable enough, but not very revealing. The following are examples of some of the fuller answers given:

'It just appeals to me more than any social work I've ever done, both for the cause itself and because here one can make an amateur contribution within a framework of professional support and advice.'

'I am not sure that I know, except that as a Christian I feel that I should give help to people if I am able to do so, and this is a sphere where service is obviously required.'

'I would like eventually to apply for the Home Office Probation Course, but would like to gain useful experience before doing so.'

'This is a field of social work that not many people would like to undertake. For me it is an interesting and challenging task.'

'Because I firmly believe that what an offender needs is someone who will seek to find and encourage that which is best in him and continue to do so in spite of disappointments and apparent failure.'

'I want to contribute to the process of taking the community into prison, and of helping the offender back into the community as I believe this is a Christian, a constructive, and a responsible way of protecting society.'

As a further attempt to obtain information about the voluntary associates' motives a question was included in the questionnaire.

Nine factors were listed all of which had, at some time, been given as a reason for wishing to become a voluntary associate. Respondents were asked to select the one which was most important to them. Inevitably this did not reflect the subtle interaction of motives. Some declined to tick only one factor. However, the answers given in Table 2 give some indication as to the relative weight of various factors.

The most striking point in Table 2 is that 'To practise their Christian beliefs' was far more frequently selected than any other single factor.

Another item in the questionnaire elicited further information about the voluntary associate's interests in professional social work. He was asked whether at any time he had applied to become a probation officer, another type of professional social worker, or a member of prison or borstal staff. He was also asked whether he anticipated any such applications in the future (see Table 3).

Of 5 (4·2 per cent) who applied for probation training since becoming voluntary associates one was accepted. A further voluntary associate became a temporary probation officer.

It is hoped that this chapter will provide some pointers to facilitate more systematic and sophisticated studies of motivation, in relation to the voluntary associates' work with clients.

TABLE 2

Primary Reason Given for Becoming a Voluntary Associate

	%
To practise their Christian beliefs	33·9
Through meeting or learning about an offender	9·1
To compensate for their daily work	7·4
As a step towards professional social work	6·6
As a substitute for not being a professional social worker	6·6
To repay good fortune in life	6·6
More than one answer	6·6
To practise their political beliefs	5·8
To fill a gap in their own interests or family life	4·2
To try to reform the penal system	4·2
Other	7·4
Don't know	1·6
N = 121	100·0

TABLE 3

Aspiration of Voluntary Associates to enter Professional Social Work

Applications Made:	Probation Officer %	Other Professional Social Worker %
Before becoming a voluntary associate*	14·0**	10·8
Since becoming a voluntary associate	4·2	1·6
Planned for the future	6·6	4·9
None	74·4	77·8
No information	0·8	4·9
	100·0	100·0
N = 121		

* Includes those with previous professional experience in social work.
** Two have re-applied since becoming voluntary associates.
   (Only 3 expressed any interest in work in the prison service.)

CHAPTER 5

TRAINING

Two Objections

There is a school of thought which argues that to train a voluntary associate is to damage his spontaneity as an ordinary citizen and to encourage him to copy the probation officer's way of working. The same school tends to stress that the relationship between voluntary associate and client should be an ordinary friendship.

There are also those who object to the word 'training' using instead 'preparation', 'induction', 'orientation', or 'briefing'. 'Training', they argue, should be reserved for the professional and implies a length and intensity inappropriate for the voluntary associate. It is however in regular use for magistrates, marriage guidance counsellors and others who undertake responsible work in a lay capacity. It is an appropriate word to describe the total process of learning, whereas terms such as 'preparation' clearly refer only to the initial stage. In the following discussion, the initial courses are described as preparation courses while the word 'training' is used to describe the total process of learning, both initially on the course and subsequently from the discussion of practical experience.

Why Training?

Critics of training have sometimes suggested that it 'contaminates' the amateur with the thoughts and habits of the professional. It is a point of view that assumes that the new voluntary associate is strangely free from prejudices, fears and misconceptions widely held by the public about ex-prisoners. Many of his attitudes and responses, like those of the general public, may be destructive, perhaps rejecting, and some facilitation of insight, so that habitual responses are understood and modified, need not be inconsistent with the role of voluntary associate. With the best of intentions the inexperienced voluntary associate frequently wants to do as much as possible for the client, perhaps to satisfy his own need to feel that he is helping. This can prompt unnecessary dependence rather than enabling the client to help himself, while the voluntary associate adopts a more supportive and passive role. Other voluntary associates may be given to moralizing, or be inclined to reject the client when problems become too great. All these, and many others, are faults which can harm the client, and are ones which can usually be modified with training. On the other hand voluntary associates have other natural qualities which can be encouraged so that they use them with greater freedom and sensitivity.

The critics of training are also adopting a point of view which would have the voluntary associate react to the ex-prisoner as if he were no different from anyone else. The intention is undoubtedly good, but it is mistaken and sometimes dangerous as Morrell[1] has explained:

'In order to establish that he is really worthy of help, some workers in the field of after-care seem impelled to "white-wash" the ex-prisoner. They refuse to see him as he really is—"warts and all". It is as though to accept him with all his limitations and personality defects is in some way inhibited by a resistance within themselves. They are prepared to help him, though perhaps not consciously, only on terms dictated by their own inner needs, involving a considerable distortion of reality, as the person is not accepted as he really is but as the worker would like him to be before he can feel completely free to help.'

Training for voluntary associates is essential, but if it is modelled too closely on that for professional social workers, its effects may be to produce a series of pale shadows of probation officers. If, on the other hand, the distinctive contribution of the voluntary associate is constantly remembered this danger can be avoided. One of the hazards for the teacher is that he, as a trained probation officer and sometimes with experience of tutoring trainee probation officers, may carry over experience gained in other situations to a type of training where they are only partly applicable. More subtly, the students may identify themselves with the teacher, modelling their subsequent work on what they think that he would have done. There is also the temptation for the teacher to be carried away into discussions which may be stimulating to some students, but confusing to others, causing them to undervalue their own less intellectually sophisticated contribution.

The experience of the project, however, showed clearly that voluntary associates needed and welcomed training. In answer to the questionnaire, no less than 80 said that they regarded the preparation course as essential and a further 38 that it was useful but not essential. Only one, who had experience as a voluntary associate before attending the course, said that it made no difference.

Training seemed to help them to see their own contribution, its relationship to that of the probation officer, and to recognize their own resources as well as their limitations. Although the project provided a longer and more systematic preparation course than many other such projects, the effect was invariably to make students aware of the extent of their ignorance and hence eager to learn more from experience and from consultation with the probation officers.

Advice from the Reports

Both the A C T O Report[2] and the Second Reading Report[3] included advice on training. The former said:

'As to training, it is necessary to stress that this is not work for inexperienced amateurs. It requires a warm heart but also a clear head, compassion combined with insight, lack of illusion, and the preparedness for disappointment. Most after-care auxiliaries will find their good intentions more effectively translated into rewarding achievement if they can have some training. . . .'

Similarly, the Second Reading Report said:

'It is generally accepted that volunteers need to be given some preparation to equip them for the tasks they will be asked to perform. . . .'

'Accredited associates, who will be undertaking long-term work with clients, will need a wider knowledge of the workings of the social services, especially the probation service, and a deeper insight into the needs of offenders and the special contribution of associates in meeting them. The probation officer selected to give this preparation should have a special interest in volunteers and an ability to teach.'

THE PREPARATION COURSE

Aims

The aims of the preparation course run by Teamwork Associates were defined as being to help the voluntary associate understand:

1. The experience, feelings, problems and needs of offenders both before and after discharge.
2. The attitudes and behaviour of the community toward the offender, and the resources of the community to help him.
3. The role of the voluntary associate, his motives and his resources.
4. The nature and significance of his relationship with the offender.
5. The voluntary associate's responsibility to the agency (the Probation and After-Care Service) and the support that he could receive from it.

Content
Under these five headings it is possible to examine the content which was included in the courses:

1. *The Offender*
Some awareness of the significance of social backgrounds of offenders and of their earlier experience in childhood seemed helpful although this had to be limited to discussion based upon cases to avoid being caught up in complex theories of causation and aetiology. More important it seemed, was the need for the students to understand how different offenders feel toward the police, the courts and the penal system. Students needed to learn not only about prison but also about the various ways in which it affects inmates and how some become 'institutionalized'. Leading on from this, it was possible to consider the various reactions and problems of the offenders on discharge, and their feelings about this.

2. *The Community*
In thinking about the offender, the attitudes and behaviour of the community toward him were also considered. The students could see themselves as members of the community and examine public feelings and attitudes towards crime and the treatment of offenders. They could also begin to look at the obligations on the community to accept the offender back and to aid the process of his reintegration.

3. *The Voluntary Associate*
The primary concern of most students was to find out what was expected of them if they became voluntary associates. Some sought more clear-cut guidance on this than it was possible to give. At the same time they were prompted to examine their own resources to help, and to measure themselves against the demands of the job. This led easily to the discussion of motives. In earlier courses a separate session was included during which students were invited to examine their motives. In later courses this was left to arise in discussion. Most students recognized it as a matter of some significance.

4. *The Relationship*
Most of the students were anxious about the kind of relationship that they might establish with a client. They needed some reassurance as to the potential value of the relationship. They also needed to understand something of the meaning of acceptance and to be forewarned about

the possibility of rejection by the client, or alternatively the demands of over-dependence, manipulation and testing out. They had to think about how far they would be prepared to go in a given situation, how much of their time they were willing to give, and how far they would involve their family or their home in the work.

5. The Agency

Normally the agency with which the voluntary associate was to work was the Probation and After-Care Service, but where an offender was still imprisoned the Prison Service was also involved. The student needed a basic appreciation of the purposes for which these services existed and the methods that they used. It was also necessary to show how Teamwork Associates, as a voluntary organization, fitted in with these statutory services. To help the students work out their relationship with the Probation and After-Care Service a short paper entitled 'Guidelines for Voluntary Associates' was prepared. This dealt with questions of accountability to the Probation and After-Care Service, its role in supporting them, and questions of ethical standards, including the clients' right to self-determination and confidentiality.

Method

A variety of teaching methods were employed. There were at least five or six lectures during each course with time for questions (see Appendix for a typical programme). Usually lectures were followed by discussions in small groups. In these groups students studied case material which gave them some insight into the problems and needs of clients in anticipation of actually meeting them.

On one evening a panel of visitors answered questions about after-care. This usually comprised a prison welfare officer, a probation officer dealing with after-care for the homeless, and one working with those returning to a settled address. Similarly experienced voluntary associates were invited to visit the course to answer questions about their work either as a panel for the whole meeting or individually in the small groups.

Early in most courses a visit of observation to one of the London prisons was arranged. Students were also given a booklist at the beginning of the course.

Length of the Course

Although some of the earliest courses extended over twelve evenings on successive weeks, the majority were about seven evenings.

Knowledge about the Social Services

Despite the advice of the second Reading Report, no attempt was made to include information about the social services, other than passing references to the Ministry of Social Security and the Ministry of Labour. To have done more would have required a further series of evenings and it was thought that voluntary associates, who would be working closely with probation officers, could draw upon their knowledge of these services when it was necessary.

Size

During the course the tutors (the director and one or two probation officers) sought to cultivate a warm, friendly and informal atmosphere. This was much easier in small courses where tutors could get to know students on a personal basis. Experience suggested that 20 to 24 students was the optimum, breaking down into two or three small groups. Less than 20 tended to lack vitality and looked depleted if members dropped out.

Anxiety

Inevitably these preparation courses tended to engender some anxiety as students began to measure themselves against the demands of the job. Every effort was made to avoid arousing additional anxiety, but to acknowledge that it was a natural response. Often it would have been easy to provoke heart-searching introspection, but this was resisted by the tutors in the belief that the experience of being a voluntary associate would facilitate the development of self-awareness gradually and at a pace with which members could cope.

At the beginning and towards the end of the course, an invitation to talk privately with one of the tutors was given. Sometimes these interviews revealed underlying problems, but no great difficulty was experienced in drawing a line between a superficial discussion and involvement in what could have become a casework relationship.

The Effectiveness of the Course

It is difficult to evaluate the effectiveness of these courses. Undoubtedly the quality of teaching improved with experience and growing confidence. Speakers became more sensitive to the reactions of their listeners, but there remained scope for imaginative use of new teaching methods and for experiments in the basic structure of courses.

The majority of the members seemed to find the course a satisfying experience. In the questionnaire those who had become voluntary associates were invited to make suggestions as to how the preparation course might have been improved in the light of their subsequent experience. The following are a selection of the suggestions:

'More talks with voluntary associates already accredited, who can talk of their personal experiences.'
'More details of statutory welfare agencies and benefits.'
'More discussion of case histories.'
'A greater degree of training—courses in psychology and sociology.'

These, and similar comments, amounted to pressure for more and, therefore, longer preparation courses.

Some requests for additional preparation were a direct reflection of the voluntary associate's subsequent experience. Thus one who had coped with a drug addict, thought that information about drug addiction should have been included in the course. Similarly one who had had a succession of disappointments thought that there should have been more 'preparation for failure'.

Perhaps the main value of the courses lay in the opportunity to examine feelings and attitudes rather than in giving information. There was also a chance to get to know a number of probation officers, to begin to work with them and to learn about their service. At the same time, the organization of the courses into small groups with a probation officer in each, and the encouragement of frank and honest discussion, was an initiation into the working methods of the project.

Details of Courses
Basic information about the starting date, length and size of each course is given in Appendix Table B, which also shows how the courses became more frequent and shorter as the project went on. The largest courses were during the second year at the time of most rapid recruitment.

REFERENCES
1. Leslie Morrell, 'The Voluntary Worker's Problems in Prison After-Care', *British Journal of Criminology*, Vol. 7 No. 4, October 1967.
2. Op. cit., par. 132.
3. Op. cit., pars. 36–45.

CHAPTER 6

SELECTION

Although Teamwork Associates allocated a substantial part of its resources to the development of preparation courses, the method of selection was regarded as even more important. Only a limited change in attitude and behaviour could reasonably be expected as a result of perhaps some fourteen hours of study. It was, then, advisable to put great reliance upon the experience, insights, knowledge and skills that the candidates brought from other spheres.

But to stress that selection was important was much easier than to devise effective methods and criteria. Advice from the official reports was limited. The ACTO Report[1] said that they wished 'to stress the importance of careful selection'; the second Reading Report[2] saw strong reasons why probation committees should accredit their own voluntary associates but did not advise as to how selection might be done, except in referring to the practice of some probation committees which required candidates to attend a preparation course as part of the selection and appointment process.

Selection for most kinds of paid employment can be based upon a job specification which can be defined in concrete terms, thus making it possible to enumerate the aptitudes and skills required. Possession of a certain standard of intelligence or education, the requisite paper qualifications and relevant experience provides a series of guidelines. In the selection of the voluntary associate there are no such basic guides.

Without a job specification it was necessary to develop methods and criteria for selection on the basis of the more general appreciation of the role of the voluntary associate (see p. 136). Once again it must be remembered that this role was capable of a wide range of interpretations. Its boundaries were constantly stretched in the light of what candidates had to offer, as much as by the needs of the clients referred.

Even after three years, during which 204 candidates were considered, it would be premature to draw firm conclusions about the best methods and criteria for selection. Over-rigid selection could inhibit the development of the role of the voluntary associate in a way which would restrict the pioneering and exploratory contribution of the voluntary movement.

It was agreed at the beginning of the project that any attempt, at that stage, to define even provisional criteria for selection would be suspect. These would have to be elicited in the light of experience. It was, however, decided that a consistent method for selection could be tested.

The Initial Interview
Those members of the public who learned about the project and made enquiries were usually invited to meet the director (or sometimes a colleague). The main purpose of each interview was to give the enquirer some basic information about the work of a voluntary associate and the aims of Teamwork Associates. The enquirer was given some idea of what would be expected of him, and some awareness of the demands, difficulties and disappointments inherent in the work. Those who were clearly not able to make a tangible offer of service could be dissuaded or encouraged to consider more appropriate forms of voluntary service. Initially no effort was made to detect those who were grossly unsuitable, but failure to do so led to several people enrolling for courses who proved disruptive or unable to participate profitably. They tended not to be aware of their own unsuitability, even at the end of the course, and were probably hurt more by ultimate rejection than other candidates who were turned down. In view of this, an effort was made later to pick out any severely psychologically sick members at the initial interview.

No records were kept of the number of enquirers and indeed it would be difficult to define what constituted an enquiry as many letters were received, without offers of interviews being taken up. But the general impression was that rather more than half of those who contacted the project enrolled for a preparation course. Readiness to attend a course was of itself a test of the enquirer's recognition of his need to learn and also of his humility. In fact, only a handful of people withdrew because of the insistence that they attend a course.

Where leaflets had been distributed widely to publicize a particular course the influx of last-minute enquirers made it impossible to interview all of them. In these circumstances it was necessary to rely upon the recommendations of other agencies or individuals, or a quick glance at the enrolment form. This was unsatisfactory for three reasons: the enquirer often had insufficient idea of what the job entailed and was more likely to take up a place on a course without subsequently offering his services; his attitude to the course tended to be more casual; and staff had no opportunity to dissuade those who seemed certain to prove unsuitable.

Self-Selection during the Course

Those who were accepted for a preparation course attended without any obligation to become voluntary associates. Similarly, Teamwork Associates was under no obligation to accept their offer of service. Although each course might have been compressed into one or two intensive weekends, it was deliberately spread out over several weeks. One object of this was to give students time for second thoughts, and for any impetuous burst of enthusiasm to wear off.

The content of the course, as we have noted, was designed to include a realistic impression of what the candidate was letting himself in for. This required that the tutors retain a balance between alarmist descriptions of the hazards and a dishonest denial of the stresses experienced by not a few voluntary associates.

During the course, tutors, especially in their small groups, had an opportunity to observe the attitudes and behaviour of students. Relationships with each other could be revealing, as could evidence of prejudice towards certain types of offender described in case studies. Regularity of attendance and time of arrival were sometimes clues as to dependability. It would, however, have been quite wrong to turn the course into a prolonged selection procedure, thus damaging the relationship between tutors and students and detracting from the learning experience.

At the penultimate meeting of each course, students were invited to make an application if they so wished. Application forms were put on a table at the front of the meeting, not distributed to students, and they were invited to complete one. A general comment was made about their help being needed, but this was never pressing, and approaches to individuals were avoided. Anyone unsure about whether to apply was invited to ask one of the tutors for an interview. On average (see Appendix Table B) about half the students made an application.

References

Two referees were always taken up. Their value lay not so much in the positive commendation of many candidates, but in the occasional warning about problems which had not previously been observed.

Selection Panels

Each candidate was then interviewed for approximately half an hour by a selection panel which consisted of a member of the project committee and a probation officer, who was usually of senior rank. Thus both voluntary and statutory partners in the work were represented. It seemed helpful to have a man and a woman on the panel, although this was not always possible. The director (or a project officer for the Youth Resettlement Project) attended most interviews but took a passive part. The probation officer, as representative of the 'employing' service, had the right to veto a candidate, although in practice the two selectors always reached an agreed decision.

Some formality was preserved in the form of the interview and candidates, on occasions, commented on its rigour. On the other hand, probation officers and other professional members of the panels were conscious of the need to set limits on their probing and to foster a warm and understanding atmosphere.

Informing Candidates

Accepted candidates received a letter of welcome from the director, enclosing a formal letter of accreditation for a probationary period of six months. This was renewable on the recommendation of the voluntary associate's consultant probation officer without further interview.

Candidates who were not accepted received a brief letter expressing regret and trying to soften the blow, but no explanation was given for the decision. Where it was appropriate, every effort was made to redirect a candidate into a more suitable, and perhaps less demanding, sphere of voluntary service. One way of doing this was to invite them to consult the Voluntary Workers Bureau at a Council of Social Service.

The Problem of Rejection

Although only 19 per cent of applicants were rejected by selection panels, it nevertheless created considerable disappointment and sometimes resentment. Time and money had been spent apparently to no avail. Perhaps more important, many candidates had made an emotional investment in the course and already felt identified with the work and with Teamwork Associates. Sometimes a candidate could be persuaded to withdraw during the interview or the panel skilfully helped him to see in advance that he would be turned down, and perhaps why, but selectors and staff alike were continually aware of the personal distress caused to some. Unlike applicants for a paid position, where there is normally only one post to be filled, candidates knew that many more voluntary associates were needed, but that they were still not acceptable.

Only by selecting before the preparation course could this kind of difficulty have been avoided, but neither selectors nor staff thought that they could have done this without the benefit of the candidates' self-selection, the observations of the tutors during the course, and the reactions of candidates to the course. Perhaps with greater experience it would be possible to select before the course, but it is doubtful whether this would be acceptable to most candidates. On one course, by way of experiment, members were invited to apply at any stage of their choosing, but almost all waited until the end. Similarly the idea of a two-part course, with selection slotted in the middle was found to be impracticable because the time needed to take up references and arrange panels led to a disruption of the training programme.

Some Relevant Factors

So far in this chapter only the method of selection has been considered. Before turning to the more difficult problem of criteria, it may be helpful to consider some of the areas in which selectors frequently asked questions.

Motivation

The candidate was often asked how he had heard about the work and what had prompted his interest. Comments gleaned from their responses have already been incorporated in Chapter 4, although many found such questions hard to answer.

Resources

Of prime importance was what the candidate was offering by way of service and whether this was usable within the terms of the project. Sometimes a candidate's resources, particularly of time, already seemed overstretched, and this might lead to neglect of family responsibilities, for example, in the case of a woman with young children. Certain practical points also shed some light on what he had to offer—willingness to travel to distant prisons, availability of his own transport, the possibility of inviting clients to his home, etc. While none of these were vital in themselves together they gave a picture which revealed whether he was making a tangible offer of service.

Relationships

The ability to form secure and warm relationships was obviously vital, as was willingness to enter into demanding relationships. Sometimes there were signs of a half-concealed reluctance to get involved, shown by limiting what was offered, in order to court rejection by the panel. At the other extreme lay the dangers of over-involvement and losing perspective, yet the need for empathy with the client.

Maturity

A high standard of maturity was obviously needed. This had several aspects: realistic expectations about what can be achieved, the ability to accept failure and yet to go on, the willingness to examine one's own feelings, to learn from experience and to submit to the observations of fellow voluntary associates and probation officers. This involved the flexibility needed to permit change, in other words was the applicant secure enough to put himself at risk in a situation which might change him as much, if not more, than it might change the client?

Authority

Since he would be working with those in authority, it was important to decide whether the candidate was likely to identify strongly for or against authority, or could preserve a balance. This necessitated an acceptance of the authority of law and the broad lines of its administration, yet recognition of the fallibility of the system and of those who operate it. At a practical level the selectors had to be sure that he could operate within a project which was closely identified with a statutory authority and with professional workers invested with a legal authority.

Values

Equally important was whether he had a firmly held moral code with the strength to maintain his own standards yet not to impose them on others. In particular, had he a sense of primary obligation to his family, or could his work as a voluntary associate upset his marriage or his private life in other ways?

Support

Lastly, the selectors were often concerned that the candidate had the full support of wife or husband (or parents) in undertaking the voluntary associate work and, if not, that alternative sources of support were available. This tied in with the need for a satisfying and full life necessary to retain balance and perspective.

Lest the reader should assume that only saints were accepted, it should be stressed that the above is an attempt to describe relevant areas of questioning, not a set of criteria. In fact, the list is far from exhaustive and even omits the oft-quoted need for a sense of humour! Not all the selectors paid equal attention to all the above and each would have added others.

Some Less Relevant Factors

It may be useful to mention some of the factors which seemed less relevant than they do in many other selection procedures. Intelligence and education did not figure much in the discussion of candidates, although a basic level was required in both. Occupation was only of interest insofar as it helped in understanding the candidate and possibly his motive in wishing to be a voluntary associate. Similarly, social class did not seem as relevant as has sometimes been suggested but selectors had to be ready to adjust in assessing those whose social background differed appreciably from their own. Previous experience in voluntary social service was not regarded as vital. Although some candidates had a wide range of experience, others had none and perhaps approached the work with fewer preconceived notions and an extra willingness to learn.

Selectors differed in the weight which they attached to the candidates' religious beliefs. In any case, this could not be dealt with in isolation but fell within several, and perhaps all, of the relevant factors listed.

Age and Sex

An arbitrary age limit for voluntary associates could have proved over-rigid. Maturity, rather than age, was the important factor, but it was decided that a minimum age of twenty-two years should be adopted, except in special circumstances. Twenty-two was chosen because it was the minimum age for probation officers, but it is also an age when most people have begun to settle down and almost all have completed full-time education. With the extension of the work to young offenders, the minimum age for the Youth Resettlement Project was set at twenty years so that at least some of the voluntary associates would be close in age to their clients. There may indeed by an argument for extending this further, teenager with teenager, but this would necessitate a careful reappraisal of the kind of supervision needed and might well be more successful in a group setting in which the distinction between client and volunteer was blurred. It is an area for future experiment, but with a necessary caution and concern to protect the young volunteer. No upward limit was set for voluntary associates, the oldest being seventy-five years.

In some other projects, doubt was expressed about the contribution which women voluntary associates could make. As male ex-prisoners outnumber females by approximately 35 to 1 it was felt that men were needed as voluntary associates, although women might help with the families. The latter was obviously important, but experience during the three years seemed to more than justify accepting women, especially those of mature years, to work with male offenders directly. There remained some apprehension about involving younger women, especially those who were single.

Making a Decision

On the basis of this broad consideration of the candidate, the actual decision usually hinged around two questions, one for each of the selectors. For the committee member the key question was whether he could commend the candidate to the Probation and After-Care Service in the confidence that he would be a good representative of the project to client, probation officer and prison officer alike. For the probation officer member the key question was whether he would have welcomed the candidate's help with one of his own cases and could envisage clients and situations in which he would want to call upon the candidate's help.

There was, of course, reluctance to reject a candidate and it was never done quickly or lightly. The view is sometimes expressed that every citizen has the right to serve his fellows, and therefore to be a volunteer. It is a noble ideal, but one which it is dangerous to apply in a particular field which makes great demands.

Grounds for rejection were usually one or more of the following:

1. A serious danger that the candidate or his client or a third party was likely to be harmed.
2. Evidence of current personal problems which were likely to have a damaging effect upon his relationship with the client, or of past personal problems about which he had little insight or with which he had not come to terms.

3. Failure to make a tangible offer of help which was likely to be usable within the scope of the Probation and After-Care Service.
4. A primary concern for the gratification of his personal needs.
5. A need to run others' lives for them, to be directive, or to propagate religious or political beliefs without due respect for the client's wishes.

The Ex-prisoner as Voluntary Associate

On six occasions ex-prisoners made enquiries about becoming voluntary associates. In broad principle, it seemed wrong for a project which 'preached' acceptance of the ex-prisoner to reserve the right to discriminate against him, but practical difficulties were anticipated. For example, it would not have been possible for them to visit prisons. The attitude of both prison and probation staff would probably have been unfavourable. Even when an ex-prisoner had made a good re-adjustment there might have been a risk of over-identification with the clients who, in any case, would be entitled to know the nature of the voluntary associate's background.

Of the six enquirers concerned, four had not long been out of prison or there was evidence of personal problems which would have disqualified them, regardless of their prison sentence. The remaining two had both been out of prison for many years and had made excellent re-adjustments. They seemed to have much to offer and the director was prepared to put them before a selection panel, subject to the approval of the principal probation officer. One enrolled for a course but failed to attend and the other decided not to enrol.

Selecting the Selectors

In view of the difficulties of defining more specifically the criteria for selection, and the highly subjective nature of the method used, much depended upon the skill of the selectors. Those drawn from the project committee included a company director with experience of staff selection, a principal prison psychologist, a senior prison chaplain, a prison governor, the director of Christian Teamwork, and latterly two voluntary associates. Those drawn from the Probation and After-Care Service were nearly all involved with voluntary associates and able to base their selection upon first-hand experience. In the Youth Resettlement Project, borstal governors also took part.

The choice of selectors rested with the director but no special arrangements were made for particular candidates to be seen by particular selectors.

Feedback

Only by a feedback to selectors of reports on the subsequent progress of accepted candidates would it have been possible to build in improvements and this was never attempted systematically or on any scale. Of those voluntary associates who later failed to cope with the work, most had been regarded as weaker candidates at the time of selection, but to argue from this that they should have been turned down would have been to ignore that others similarly assessed appeared to have done well. In other words, there was an area of calculated risk, which the six month probationary period provided a chance to correct.

The Ultimate Selection

The real test came when the newly accredited voluntary associate was introduced to his local team. Would he prove acceptable to his consultant probation officer and to the team? Would the probation officer and his colleagues have the confidence in him to entrust their clients to his care? Most important of all, and the ultimate selection, would the client accept him? These were the vital stages in selection at the end of a long line of hurdles which had eliminated, mainly of their own volition, the majority of starters.

The Elite?

Approximately 20 per cent of the original enquirers survived to accreditation. Selection procedures of this kind have been criticized in that they tend to deter all but the most persistent candidates, leaving an 'elite' who, by virtue of their social class and education, are more familiar with, and more tolerant of such methods. It is probably true. The justification for such methods, during the period covered by the project, lay in an acceptance of the complaint by many probation officers that the calibre of voluntary associates in the past had not always been to their satisfaction. Thus a major concern was to select voluntary associates who would win the confidence of probation officers and, if the latter are right in their assessment, prove effective and dependable in helping the clients.

REFERENCES

1. Op. cit., par. 131.
2. Op. cit., pars. 22, 23, 42.

CHAPTER 7

THE VOLUNTARY ASSOCIATES

The typical volunteer in the social services, as the Aves Committee[1] observed, is commonly thought to be a 'middle-aged, middle-class, married woman'. Its evidence suggested that there was some foundation for this belief, but showed also that such people no longer constituted an overwhelming majority among the total volunteer force. Men were playing a greater part than was sometimes realized. This would seem to be especially true in after-care.

Similarly the age range has widened. Lacey[2] (1962) said that as a general policy voluntary associates were usually not under 30 years, and not over 55 years. Of 75 voluntary associates in his sample the age distribution was as follows:

Years	%	
26–30	9·3	
31–40	28·0	
41–50	34·7	(Men 50
51–60	22·7	Women 25)
61–70	5·3	

Average age: 44·2 years.

He also noted that their occupations tended to be middle class (although they were not analysed according to the Registrar-General's classification).

The emphasis which Teamwork Associates put during the initial year on recruitment through the churches created a bias towards a predominantly middle-class sector of the community. As a result the project was not well placed to broaden the range of social class from which voluntary associates came. It was, however, possible to broaden the age range considerably, especially to explore ways in which younger people could help. Similarly, women were able to play a full part, including some who might previously have been regarded as much too young.

During the three years a total of 175 voluntary associates were accredited, of whom 20 subsequently dropped out. (Thus the actual strength at the end of the project was 155.) The data in the remainder of this chapter are taken from the enrolment forms completed by them before attending a preparation course, unless otherwise stated.

Drop-outs

In view of the opportunity for self-selection during the preparation course it was hoped that the rate of drop out after accreditation would be minimal. This proved to be so and, as the following list of reasons for withdrawal shows (Table 4), there was little evidence of inability to cope or disillusionment with the job:

TABLE 4

Reasons of Voluntary Associates for Withdrawing

Moved away from the London area	12*
Change of family circumstances	3
Accreditation not renewed after 6 months	1
Became a temporary probation officer	1
Transferred as voluntary associate to probation and after-care service nearer his home	1
Not given work by local probation officers	1
Lost contact with them—reason not known	1
	20

* Includes 2 starting full-time course in social studies. Several of these retained contact with clients by letter or occasional visits.

TABLE 5

Age of Voluntary Associates

Age	Borough teams	Percentage Withdrawals*	Youth Resettlement Project	All groups
Up to 25	19·7	35·0	39·5	25·7
26–30	20·5	40·0	18·5	22·2
31–40	23·9	5·0	36·8	24·6
41–50	19·7	10·0	2·6	14·9
51–60	11·9	10·0	2·6	9·7
61 and over	4·3	—	—	2·9
Total	100·0	100·0	100·0	100·0
N =	117	20	38	175

* All withdrawals were from Borough teams.

Age

Table 5 gives details of the age of the voluntary associates. In this table only, separate figures are given for the Youth Resettlement Project as the difference in age is appreciable.

In making any comparison between these figures for age and those given by Lacey, it is necessary to bear in mind that the latter was not using a representative sample of voluntary associates at that time. However, there can be no doubt that Teamwork Associates involved more young voluntary associates than did the earlier projects or some current ones. As Table 5 shows, 48 per cent of those associated with Teamwork Associates were 30 years or under.

The average age was 35·8 for all the voluntary associates and 29·8 for those in the Youth Resettlement Project. It will also be noted that withdrawals tended to be in the younger age groups which indicated the greater mobility of young people rather than their lack of ability to stick to the job.

Throughout the social services young volunteers have increased in number during recent years, and the same mood of idealism seemed to prompt support for the project. Unlike some earlier projects Teamwork Associates made no assumption that young people would be less useful than their elders. Similarly, there was a feeling that fears about involving women had been overplayed.

As in other fields of voluntary service, women seemed easier to recruit. Some hesitated to take up the work when they discovered that the large majority of ex-prisoners were men, and others were encouraged to take up work for offenders' families, but many of mature age and outlook were accredited to work with the men. Undoubtedly, they brought qualities to the work not shared by their male colleagues and increased the scope for matching the voluntary associate to the needs of the client (see p. 87).

The problem of younger single women was more complicated. The experience of young women as probation officers in prison welfare and after-care had done much to add an air of normality to the work, for clients and colleagues alike, and had largely overcome apprehension. But these women officers had a degree of professional protection and of training not possessed by the young woman who was a voluntary associate. For her there seemed to be a genuine risk of emotional involvement with the client which, even if she was able to understand and control it, might present an unreasonable situation for the client, who was less able to grasp the subtleties of the relationship between the voluntary associate and himself.

The difficulty was made more acute by the fact that there were frequent offers of help from young women who combined a youthful femininity with a mature concern. Given the opportunity to become voluntary associates, many of them seemed likely to become especially valuable workers at a later stage. When the Youth Resettlement Project was started it was decided that these younger women might be helpful in working with some of the younger, more immature, borstal boys, providing adequate support was available and great care was taken in selecting both parties. It is much too soon to comment on their success in this field, but initial signs are encouraging. In the meantime the presence of mini-skirted voluntary associates in the institutions has done much to change the stereotype of the volunteer for both staff and in-mates.

Marital Status

Table 6 shows the marital status of the 175 voluntary associates.

TABLE 6

Marital Status of Voluntary Associates

	%
Married	45·7
Single	49·7
Widowed, divorced or separated	4·6
N = 175	100·0

That over half the voluntary associates were single at the time of enrolment for the project, of course, partly related to the recruitment of young applicants, but there were many older ones for whom voluntary service may have offered some kind of involvement with people and means a fulfilment which others find with their families. Although some single voluntary associates tended to feel at a disadvantage they could sometimes be more mobile and give more time than someone with family commitments.

The married voluntary associates included nine husbands and wives who worked together. In addition, a number of others had husbands or wives who took an active part in the work without asking to become accredited voluntary associates. Similarly, boy friends and girl friends of the single voluntary associates sometimes took an active interest.

Occupation and Social Class

The occupations of the voluntary associates ranged from stockbroker to storekeeper and from associate television producer to plasterer. However, the majority were involved in white collar work, frequently of a professional and highly responsible kind (see Table 7).

TABLE 7

Occupations of Voluntary Associates	%
Clerical and secretarial	19.9
Engineering and scientific	10·3
Teaching	8·7
Housewives	7·9
Management and administration	6·8
Central and local government officers	5·8
Medical, dental & nursing	4·6
Full-time religious work	3·9
Social work/welfare/personnel	3·9
Barrister/solicitor	3·4
Students	2·9
Retired	2·3
Salesmen	2·3
Journalists	1·8
Television production	1·8
Other*	13·8
N = 175	100·1

* Other included jobs as various as actress, air hostess, regular soldier, RSPCA inspector, librarian and caretaker.

Using the Registrar General's classification of occupations as a means of categorizing the voluntary associates into social class groups, shows a heavy preponderance in the professional, intermediate and skilled classes (see Table 8).

TABLE 8

Social class of Voluntary Associates	%
I. Professional etc.	21·1
II. Intermediate	36·6
III. Skilled	30·3
IV. Partly skilled	1·8
V. Unskilled	0·6
Students	2·9
Housewives (not employed)	6·8
N = 175	100·1

Education

As would be expected from the above details of occupation, a large number of the voluntary associates held technical, commercial or professional qualifications and 30 were graduates.

Information about the type of school attended was taken from the 121 replies to the questionnaire.

Twenty seven per cent had attended independant schools (compared with 67 per cent in Lacey's study) and 50 per cent grammar schools. Only 14 per cent had had a secondary modern education.

TABLE 9

Type of School Attended by Voluntary Associates

	%
Independent ('public' 'private')	27·3
Grammar	49·6
Technical	3·3
Secondary Modern	14·0
Not educated in the United Kingdom	1·7
No information	4·1
N=121	100·0

If we again make a comparison with Lacey's figures we find that the proportion of voluntary associates educated at independent schools in Teamwork Associates was 27 per cent against 67 per cent in his sample.

Religion

In view of the special efforts during the project to mobilize support within the churches the religious beliefs of voluntary associates may be of interest. On their enrolment form they were asked to state whether their religion was 'active' or 'nominal' and this distinction has been recorded in Table 10.

Of those on whom information was available 57 per cent professed active religious belief of one sort or another, and they represented a wide range of religious tradition.

Geographical Distribution

Appendix Table A shows the number of voluntary associates who worked in each borough. Not all of them lived in the same borough, and 45 lived outside Inner London. There was also a tendency to live at the outer fringes of the inner boroughs, e.g. Hampstead in the Borough of Camden. It was difficult to find voluntary associates from the older twilight areas.

TABLE 10
Religious Beliefs of Voluntary Associates

	'Active'	'Nominal'	Total	%
Church of England	39	36	75	(42·9)
Roman Catholic	20	3	23	(13·1)
Free Church (Methodist, Baptist, Congregationalist)	26	3	29	(16·6)
Church of Scotland & Presbyterian	5	2	7	(4·0)
Pentecostal	3	–	3	(1·7)
Lutheran	–	2	2	(1·1)
Quaker	2	–	2	(1·1)
Jewish	3	5	8	(4·6)
Christian Science	1	–	1	(0·6)
	99	51	150	(85·7)
Humanist			2	(1·1)
Agnostic			6	(3·4)
Atheist			1	(0·6)
None			8	(4·6)
No information			8	(4·6)
			25	(14·3)
		Grand total:	175	(100·0)

Previous experience

Information was also recorded about voluntary associates' previous experience of 'voluntary social work, work with offenders, youth work, and church work' (see Table 11).

TABLE 11
Previous Experience of Voluntary Associates

	%	
Voluntary social work	50·9	
Paid social work	8·6	
Work with offenders	26·9	(percentages of
Youth work	48·6	175)
Church work	44·6	
No previous experience	17·7	

Of the total of 175 only 31 stated that they had no previous experience in any of these fields. Thus, as a group, they tended to be experienced, although its extent, its relevance and its value, varied greatly. The following are some examples:

Voluntary Social Work
Interviewer for Citizens Advice Bureau, Community Service Volunteer, Voluntary Service Overseas, International Voluntary Service Camps, work for Family Welfare Association, Marriage Guidance Counsellor.

Paid Social Work
Assistant housemaster in children's home, Welfare Officer in Royal Navy, welfare work with immigrants, residential work with alcoholics.

Work with Offenders
Retired policeman, special constable, magistrate, member of Oxford University borstal camps, member of after-care organizations, informal contact with offenders in a private capacity.

Youth Work
Warden of Youth Conference Centre, work with 'unattached' young people, youth club leaders.

Church Work
Sunday school teaching, pastoral work.

Nationality
In a cosmopolitan city some voluntary associates who were immigrants might be expected. There were in fact 13 of them (West Indians: 3, Irish: 3, Germans: 2, Austrian: 1, Danish: 1, Hungarian: 1, American: 1, Singalese: 1).

The Ordinary Citizen
On the basis of the above information it would have been impossible to describe the voluntary associates as 'ordinary citizens', but they themselves would have disclaimed any suggestion that they were an 'elite' group and seemed to attach little significance to paper qualifications of the sort recorded on an enrolment form. Warmth, understanding, tolerance and commitment were not so easily measured, but it was such qualities as these which seemed important.

We shall discuss later the issue of social class touched upon in this chapter. However, we must, at this stage, record the feelings of the voluntary associate about this issue. Many of them resisted any labelling in class terms and attention given to the matter in this report is a response to the importance sometimes attached to it by others outside the project and not a reflection of its importance internally. While anxieties about differences of background, or having the wrong accent, were sometimes expressed on preparation courses, they were rarely repeated on the job, and seemed to be a focus for 'beginners' nerves' rather than a major obstacle. Whatever pen picture of the typical voluntary associate emerges from this chapter, and generalizations are almost certainly misleading, they clearly looked upon themselves as just ordinary people and this self concept was perhaps their greatest strength.

REFERENCES

1. Op. cit., par. 37.
2. Op. cit.

CHAPTER 8

THE CLIENTS

Source of Information
Information about the clients introduced to voluntary associates has been taken from the probation officers' case records. It is, therefore, limited to those factors which had been recorded for administrative and casework purposes. For research purposes it would have been preferable to ask the probation officer to complete special schedules on each of these clients, but this would have been a heavy burden on people who were already working under pressure and giving their time generously to support the project. The additional paper work could have deterred officers from referring cases to the voluntary associates.

Instead the probation officers were asked to complete a short return on each client referred so that further information could be gleaned from the official case record in due course. The returns were usually, but not invariably, completed. As a further source of information the voluntary associates were asked in the questionnaire for the names of their clients, and, where additional cases came to light, the probation officer was asked for full details. By this method information was received on a total of 237 clients. Further cross-checking revealed some missed cases especially during the first two years of the project. If the probation officer and/or the voluntary associate had moved, cases were difficult to trace. There also seemed to be tendency to forget cases which 'never got off the ground' or where contact ceased after only one or two meetings. But the 237 cases on which information was obtained undoubtedly represent the vast majority of referrals from probation or welfare officers to voluntary associates during the 3 years.

Unfortunately the records on these cases were not all completed equally thoroughly, and the general standard for after-care was poorer than for probation. Details of work with prisoners' families was often not recorded. In view of these deficiencies information needed on each case was sometimes incomplete.

In addition to these 237 cases a further 22 were known to be in touch with voluntary associates, but had not been referred by probation or welfare officers. Some had been in touch with the voluntary associate before they had joined the project; others had made direct contact. Many of these cases were discussed regularly at team meetings and with probation officers.

Voluntary associates also undertook specific short-term tasks from time to time—a single visit to a family, collecting luggage, providing an unofficial 'escort' across London etc. Records of such work were not kept.

In general, the availability of voluntary associates tended to be just ahead of the development of sufficient interest by probation officers to start making referrals. Thus there was some 'slack' especially in new teams, but this seemed to be a teething trouble rather than a permanent problem. Latterly in some boroughs the demand for voluntary associates began to outstrip supply. In general, however, the resources of the project were never put under pressure. While the close working partnership with probation officers encouraged more referrals than to some other organizations, the development of confidence was slow.

The contribution of the voluntary associates must not, of course, be measured solely in terms of their work during the project. Most of them seem likely to continue in the work over a long period and their total 'productivity' may be substantial, especially when the intensive and long-term nature of the relationships with clients is recognized. The pilot project can be seen as a time of preparation for this future service.

Referrals to Each Team
Appendix Table C, shows the number of referrals to each of the borough teams and to the Youth Resettlement Project. Variations were partly explained by the different size of teams and by the length of contact established with each client, but there were also differences in pressure of work.

Types of Referral
Early in the project referrals were almost exclusively prison after-care cases, but the range began to widen once the borough teams were established. Two explanations can be given for this. First, the amount of on-going after-care work done in the boroughs varied considerably. After-care work for the voluntary associates was not forthcoming on

the scale anticipated and the development of voluntary services along-side the probation officers was perhaps premature. Second, there seemed no need to confine the voluntary associates rigidly to after-care and it was considered that there might be value in experimenting with intro-ductions to other types of client (see Appendix Table D). It was during the second year that this suggestion began to be taken up.

In addition to the Youth Resettlement Project, several of the borough teams accepted the referral of homeless borstal boys. Once voluntary associates had been introduced to prisoners and to borstal boys on licence, it was only a short step to referring probationers. Parole was not operative on any scale during the project, but towards the end it became clear that a number of parolees were likely to be referred. The involvement with prisoners' families reflected a growing concern to help them in response to criticism that their needs had not been fully recognized or met in the past.

The referral of matrimonial cases to voluntary associates should not be mistaken for a form of marriage-guidance counselling. These were cases where the need for support, either for the family or for a separated party, had become evident to the probation officer in the course of his efforts to effect reconciliation.

The wide field in which the voluntary associates were involved can be seen as a welcome development, providing it does not detract from the need to improve services for the prisoner and ex-prisoner.

Referrals from Institutions
About half the referrals from prisons came from welfare officers and the other half from liaison probation officers. Some of these referrals, espec-ially from welfare officers, were made via the director, but several borough teams began to establish links with particular prisons and to obtain direct requests. These were often regarding homeless men who did not have any ties with the borough in question. Referrals of borstal boys were usually from liaison probation officers. The numbers referred from each prison, borstal or other institution are given in Appendix Table E.

It will be noted that many of these institutions were far from London, but voluntary associates showed a commendable willingness to travel and to make regular visits before discharge. The number of referrals from London prisons was fewer than had been hoped, in view of their size and the number of inmates from Inner London. However, those which had a substantial number of discharges locally (Pentonville,

Wandsworth and Holloway) already had well-developed links with other voluntary organizations. While there were undoubtedly more inmates who might have been referred, the welfare officers were working under heavy pressure with serious staff shortages.[1] In contrast smaller prisons outside London had a better ratio of welfare officers to inmates, lower turnover and more favourable working conditions.

Perhaps the most striking feature of Appendix Table E, is the wide scatter of institutions which made referrals to Teamwork Associates. Other voluntary associate projects in London tended to have more referrals from just one or two key sources.

Types of Offence
Appendix Table F, gives the principal offence for which the clients had been last convicted. Categorized in the table, the gravity of many of the offences and their great variety is not apparent. They included 3 convicted for murder, 3 for manslaughter and 3 for buggery and others for rape, drug offences, arson and possession of firearms. While the legal definition of an offence is sometimes misleading as a guide to the general characteristics of the offender, and the majority referred to the voluntary associates seemed relatively passive rather than violent, there were clearly exceptions.

Most clients had previous convictions (see Table 12) the maximum being 43.

TABLE 12
Clients' Previous Times Convicted %

None	10·5
1	7·6
2	6·3
3	8·9
4	10·5
5–10	20·3
11–20	10·9
21+	2·5
Not applicable	15·3
No information	7·2
N=237	100·0

They also tended to have had previous sentences of imprisonment or borstal training (see Table 13). Many of those technically probationers at the time of referral had been in prison or borstal previously. Thus their referral was often consistent with the original aims of the project in a way which was not immediately apparent. (Many of the borstal boys were known to have been to approved schools and some to detention centres, but such information was not always recorded for older clients.) The total length of prison or borstal sentence could not be calculated from the records, but clearly the majority had a long history of institutional confinement.

TABLE 13

Clients' previous Sentences of Imprisonment and/or Borstal Training

	%
None	32·9
I	6·8
2	5·1
3	6·3
4	2·5
5–10	13·5
11–20	4·6
21+	0·4
Not applicable	15·2
No information	12·7
N = 237	100·0

Age and Sex

Despite serious histories of offending and institutional treatment the majority were under 30 (see Table 14). Fewer women were referred as would be expected. Thirty were the wives of prisoners and their ages were very rarely recorded.

TABLE 14

Age and Sex of Clients

	Male*	Female	Total
	%	%	%
Up to 20	23·7	10·6	21·1
21–30	38·6	14·9	32·9
31–40	15·7	12·8	15·2
41–50	21·1	8·5	11·4
51–60	5·8	4·3	5·5
61 +	0·5	6·4	1·7
Not known	4·7	42·6	12·2
Total	100·1	100·1	100·0
N =	190	47	237

* Where offender and his family were clients the age of the former only has been included.

Family circumstances

The marital status of the clients is given in Table 15.

TABLE 15
Marital Status of Clients

	Male %	Female %	Total %
Single	61·2	23·4	53·6
Married	16·3	55·3	24·0
Co-habiting Living apart	4·7	8·5	5·5
Legally separated	8·4	2·1	7·2
Divorced	4·7	–	3·8
Widowed	0·5	6·4	1·7
Not known	4·2	4·3	4·2
Totals	100·0	100·0	100·0
N =	190	47	237

One hundred and fourteen (48 per cent) were described by the probation officer as homeless. No fewer than 118 (49 per cent) were said to have no relatives in the Inner London area.

Comment

Any idea that voluntary associates should deal only with the less hardened or less damaged client would not be consistent with the way in which they were actually used. The picture presented in this chapter reflects the kind of client with whom probation officers are dealing in Inner London since the extension of their duties to include the 'hard core' of offenders. Probation officers seem ready to involve voluntary associates as partners in this difficult work, where the prognosis is often poor, rather than on the periphery of their duties with less damaged and perhaps more hopeful cases. This could be interpreted as unloading the most impossible clients on to the unsuspecting voluntary associate. From time to time this may have happened, but the frequency with which probation officers and voluntary associates shared the case (p. 99) suggests that the former was prompted not by the need to unload but to spread the load.

REFERENCE

1. *Social Work in Prison,* Report of London Branch of the National Association of Probation Officers, 1969.

CHAPTER 9

MATCHING

Much has been said about the importance of matching voluntary associate and client, but very little about how this should actually be done. The second Reading Report[1] said:

'Systematic attempts to match associates to offenders have been few, there is little evidence of success and no doubt the complexities of human nature will ensure that the art remains imprecise.'

Certainly matching is an art rather than science, but the experience of the project suggests that it is crucially important however difficult.

Why Attempt to Match?
In the field of professional social work, experiments have been conducted to match the needs of the clients to types of treatment given by workers with specific skills. In the delinquency field the best known of these is the California Community Treatment Project.[2] In the United Kingdom the Probation Research Project[3] has revealed differences in the treatment emphases of probation officers and a small-scale experiment in matching probation officer and probationer has been attempted in Sheffield, but no results are, so far, published.[4]

However, there tends to be an assumption that the professional, as a result of his training, can adapt his style of work and treatment methods in response to the varying needs of the clients. For the voluntary associate, the opposite assumption is sometimes made, namely that he is likely to have a restricted range of responses to the clients' needs. Therefore, it is argued, it is necessary to ensure that he is introduced to clients able to benefit from what he has to offer. If this distinction is valid, then it follows that matching is more important for the voluntary associate than for the probation officer.

Any attempt at the beginning of the project to lay down guidelines for matching was impossible in the absence of any relevant experience or evidence. Three methods were tried of which the third was by far the most common. They might be given the names 'spontaneous', 'responsive' and 'contrived'.

Spontaneous Matching

Spontaneous matching involves the creation of a social situation in which a number of clients and voluntary associates can interact freely, so that a natural process of pairing can take place on the basis of mutual attraction. The Shepton Mallett Project demonstrated how this could be done within a prison by free association between inmates and visiting voluntary associates.

The advantage of this form of matching is that it relieves the probation officers of an extremely difficult task, and involves the client and the voluntary associate in a free choice in circumstances akin to those in which relationships are established in other aspects of life. But it cannot be assumed that this process of 'natural selection' will necessarily accord with the needs of the client, as seen by the probation officer. It may rather be a way of satisfying his wants which may or may not be the same as his needs. There are risks, especially with the demanding or manipulative client who selects a voluntary associate who seems to be open to exploitation. However, hazards of this sort can be avoided if both clients and voluntary associates are selected for the meetings, which implies a form of generalized matching leaving an element of free choice. A further practical difficulty is that the number of settings in which spontaneous matching can take place are limited. Thus it remains a method which has not yet been fully explored.

Responsive Matching

A second method which retains an element of choice by one party might be called responsive matching. This was tried by some of the borough teams and again relieved the probation officer of some of the difficulties of matching. The method was quite simply to outline the problems and needs of a new case to the team and to invite members to discuss it with a view to deciding whether a voluntary associate could help and, if so, whether one of them would volunteer to do so.

In the course of such a discussion some members would 'warm' to the case and begin to feel that they could help. The team could then discuss which of the members who were responsive to the request for help could take on additional work at that stage and which would be best suited to meet the client's needs.

Contrived Matching

The most frequent method of matching was contrived matching in which the consultant probation officer took the full responsibility for selecting the appropriate voluntary associate for the client. At first this task seemed daunting and the notion that one should contrive to bring about 'a friendship' was hard to accept. But as the role of the voluntary associate became more clearly defined, and he began to be seen less as the ordinary friend, so it became possible to look at matching in terms of a treatment or after-care plan for the client.

Basically the task could be seen in one of two ways: either some attempt could be made to match the needs of the client with the resources of the voluntary associate, or an attempt could be made to match the expectations of the client and the voluntary associate in terms of what each was wanting from the relationship and had to offer to it. In practice, most matchings tended to be based primarily on the former, but it was usual to give each party at least a thumb nail sketch of the other so that they had a chance to decline. The voluntary associate was never pressed to accept a case and it was not uncommon for him to decline.

Some voluntary associates expressed clear preferences for work, for example, with younger offenders or with 'those for whom there seemed to be some hope'. Personal inclinations of this sort were usually discussed at their selection interview and later with their consultant probation officer. One advantage of working in small teams was that the consultant got to know his members, their interests, attitudes and prejudices, so that he was able to attempt a more sophisticated matching than would have been possible for the director, who could not hope to know over a hundred voluntary associates well. But a small team could offer only a limited choice and frequently only one or two members were available to take a new client at the appropriate moment. In these circumstances matching was hardly applicable.

Sometimes such difficulties were overcome by reference to the director, or to a neighbouring team, so that a suitable voluntary associate might be found. This was also important if a request arose for a voluntary associate with some specific skill. But there was a general reluctance to beg and borrow from one team to another, partly because this led to complications regarding supervision.

Factors Thought to be Relevant in Matching

The following factors were those most frequently considered in matching:

Common Interests or Leisure Activities

These seemed important where it was hoped that the voluntary associate could be companion or a means of introducing the client into a community.

Age and Sex

Sometimes the primary need seemed to be for a relationship with someone who could compensate for past or current deficiencies in the client's relationships. Thus he might seem to need a mother figure, or a father figure. Similarly he might seem to need a relationship with someone close to his own age as a step towards better relationships with his peers. In the case of immature young clients, a relationship with a female voluntary associate who was not very much older sometimes seemed to be helpful in gaining confidence in the company of the opposite sex.

In Table 16 the sex of both the clients and the voluntary associates are given, showing how they were matched. Female clients included family situations where the wife was involved without her husband. Where the husband was also involved the case has been recorded as Male/Female. Where the voluntary associate is shown as Male/Female this was often, though not always, a married couple working together.

TABLE 16

Matching of Clients and Voluntary Associates by Sex

| | *Voluntary Associates* | | | |
Clients	Male	Female	Male and Female	Total
Male	106	55	20	181
Female	1	43	3	47
Male and Female	1	7	1	9
Total	108	105	24	237

It will be noted that only once was a male voluntary associate used on his own with a female client and this was a family situation. This reflected the normal, though not universal, practice of probation officers.

In Table 17 the similarity or difference in age between client and voluntary associate are compared for 177 relationships for which the necessary information was available on both parties. For this purpose couples were excluded.

TABLE 17

Age Comparison of Clients and Voluntary Associates

	Both Male %	Both Female %	Female Vol. Associate Male Client %	Totals %
Voluntary associate more than five years younger than client.	12·9	29·6	18·4	16·9
Not more than five years difference in age.	33·7	29·6	26·5	31·1
Voluntary associate more than five years older than client.	53·4	40·8	55·1	52·0
Totals	100·0	100·0	100·0	100·0
N =	101	27	49	177

Some Examples

The following are just a few examples of contrived matching. The first is based upon a single factor—the need for accommodation, the second on a similarity of circumstances and interest, and the third on a combination of interest, availability and the need for a mother figure:

1. A homeless borstal boy needed accommodation for home leave. He was matched with a voluntary associate who had specifically offered such help and was prepared to regard it as the start of a long-term relationship 'if things worked out'.

2. A young married couple with small children were allocated a tenth-floor flat on a new housing estate some eight miles from the old neighbourhood where they had been brought up. The husband was on probation and out of work. Both seemed depressed and lonely. Another young couple, both of whom were voluntary associates and themselves recently married, were invited to visit at the suggestion of the probation officer. They were able to baby-sit so that the first couple could get out, and to invite them to their own house. It was also possible to support the probation officer in his efforts to help the husband obtain work.

3. An immature prisoner in his twenties with a deprived childhood and no family ties asked for a voluntary associate following a group meeting when the director visited the prison. The prisoner had a keen interest in art and the welfare officer suggested that a voluntary associate was needed who shared this interest, and preferably a woman. It was possible to select as the voluntary

associate a family woman with a grown-up son and an appreciation of art. She also lived on the right side of London, and had her own transport to visit the prison, which was inaccessible and some distance away.

Matching with the Probation Officer

A further factor which the consultants began to regard as important was matching the voluntary associate with the probation officer who was already involved with the client. If the voluntary associate and the probation officer were to work well together then mutual respect was an asset. In some instances working partnerships were established so that a particular voluntary associate regularly took referrals from one probation officer.

Effectiveness of Contrived Matching

While some matchings seemed to be inspired and the two parties seemed to 'click', there were others where the relationship was less comfortable or faltered. But the ability to get on well need not always indicate that the relationship is helping to meet the client's needs; nor does a less comfortable relationship necessarily mean that it is unhelpful to the client. He may learn much through the strains and stresses of such a relationship. Breakdown in the relationship, at an early stage, was not uncommon, but it was difficult to attribute this to 'bad' matching when it might have happened in any case, or have resulted from a lack of preparation of either or both parties.

Preparing the Client

A frequent reason for breakdown in the relationship seemed to be a failure on the part of the client to understand its purpose. Naturally he tended to refer back in his mind to previous people who had shown interest in him. Sometimes, in the case of a prisoner, it might be a prison visitor. If so, he was likely to think of the voluntary associate purely as a visitor during sentence, maybe as a break in the monotony, and not as someone with whom to keep in touch after discharge. Similarly, there was a tendency to assume that the voluntary associate had deep pockets and was good for a 'soft touch', or might be manipulated into pulling strings for him—a stereotype which may have fitted some voluntary workers in the offender's past experience.

In view of these misconceptions it was clearly important to explain fully who and what the voluntary associate was, and the way in which he could or could not help. Again no guidelines were suggested to prison welfare officers and probation officers and practice obviously differed, depending upon their perception of a voluntary associate and the needs of the client. Sometimes the officer referred specifically to having 'a voluntary associate' from a voluntary organization, or to some 'friends of mine' who sometimes help the probation officers.

The thoroughness of the clients' preparation to meet the voluntary associate clearly varied. One voluntary associate commented:

> 'I should like to see a better system evolved for introducing client to voluntary associate. In my two years' experience, it seems to me that the two are thrown together with little preparation and a large percentage of clients seem very reluctant about the relationship.'

A consultant probation officer commented:

> 'The probation officer does not seem to be aware of the necessity to prepare the client for the advent of a voluntary associate and, in consequence, may try to hurry the process. The result of this can be disastrous for the voluntary associate (as well as for the client) and very disappointing if failure is experienced in the early stages.'

Obviously, probation officers dealing with an unfamiliar situation, found it difficult. The experience of the project, however, suggested that successful matching must go hand in hand with careful preparation. It may also be necessary to reassure the client that the probation officer is not rejecting him or 'passing the buck'. If the probation officer intends to retain contact as well, this needs to be said, with some comment upon any change in the frequency of meetings. If he intends to hand over, then many of the same considerations will apply as in the transfer of a client from one probation officer to another.

Preparing the Voluntary Associate

The voluntary associate also needed preparation before being introduced to the client. The probation officer had to decide how much it was helpful to tell the voluntary associate about the client. Officers varied in their practice. Some readily handed the file to the voluntary associate while others were unwilling to reveal confidential information.

Too much information, all at once, could confuse, and perhaps frighten the voluntary associate. If the official file was a long one it could not be readily digested by someone inexperienced in handling it and untrained in sifting essential from non-essential information. But, at the other extreme, reluctance to share information could be construed by the voluntary associate as a lack of trust and a lack of willingness to accept him as a partner. A minority of voluntary associates preferred not to know very much about the client, so that he could reveal himself in his own way, at his own pace, and just so much as he wished to do. This, it was felt, put the relationship on a more normal basis, but most voluntary associates felt reassured if they knew something of the offences and a little of the background before being introduced.

A rigid practice about this would be unhelpful. Again the appropriate course depends upon the wishes of both parties and the judgement of the probation officer. One point, however, is clear, that is that information about the client should not be revealed to the voluntary associate without his permission. If this is observed as an ethical principle, then it helps to put the relationship with the voluntary associate on a different footing from that with another professional worker, where his colleague would have passed on the information without asking for the client's consent. The probation officer may find, at this stage, an opportunity to explain to the client his own relationship with the voluntary associate and that from time to time he will be asking him how he (the client) is getting along. The probation officer may also, in return for permission to share information with the voluntary associate, tell the client something about him, thus introducing an element of reciprocity.

As voluntary associates have gained the respect of probation officers, so their readiness to share confidential material has increased, and the officers have known that the voluntary associates are required to accept the same level of confidentiality as professional social workers. But the freedom to share confidential information within the professional agency should not be extended beyond its boundaries without the consent of the client.

In addition to deciding how, and how much, information to pass on to the voluntary associate, the probation officer also had to describe how he hoped the voluntary associate could help. When they were to share the case there was a need to clarify their respective roles and to define the boundary between them.

A further factor to be clarified at this stage was the means of accountability by the voluntary associate to the probation officer, and the kind of circumstances in which he should get in touch.

Establishing a Standard
Some probation officers may well feel that the above proposals for preparing each party are a counsel of perfection, which cannot be maintained under normal pressures of work. Certainly it would be misleading to imply that they were always maintained during the project. They

are, however, included here because they seem vitally important if the relationship between client and voluntary associate is to stand a fair chance of getting off the ground, and if both parties are to be accorded the consideration and respect that they deserve. That this calls for a high standard of professional competence and a willingness to devote time on the part of the referring probation officer is just another indication of the demands which such work makes upon him.

REFERENCES

1. Op. cit., par. 46.
2. See E. Palmer, *An Overview of Matching in the Community Treatment Project* and other reports by same author, Department of the Youth Authority, State of California.
3. Op. cit.
4. An experiment included in the Probation Research Project of the Home Office Research Unit, report not yet published.

CHAPTER 10

THE RELATIONSHIP

Reasons for Referral

The reasons for referral given by the probation officers and the prison officers were many and varied. But the recurrent theme of their comments was the need to give support, to overcome loneliness or to give the client some sense of belonging. The following reasons were extracted from the case records:

Adult Offenders

'Lonely man, estranged from his family, ill with bronchitis—needing friendship.'

'Lonely prisoner, has difficulty in making relationships, needs a voluntary associate to keep him in touch with life outside.'

'German with poor English, living in Salvation Army Hostel. Completely isolated socially.'

'Sex offender, elderly, recently widowed. First offence of indecent assault on small boys. Devastated by conviction and imprisonment.'

'A lonely embittered man. Marriage broken up, no relatives or friends. Frequently returns to prison out of despair. Still able to relate fairly well when opportunity arises.'

Young Offenders

'An 18-year-old youth on probation, living in lodgings, mother in mental hospital, father dead. Little interest in work or leisure.'

'West Indian girl, pregnant, alone in this country—needing support.'

'Youth aged 20 in Detention Centre. Difficulty in relating to his mother and to his stepfather, who is only 18 months older. Needs substitute parents to visit and invitation to their home on discharge.'

Families

'Immigrant family. Father in prison for murdering his daughter. Wife and four children very isolated. Need for practical help as well as friendly support.'

'Miss B and her three children are returning from a Family Rehabilitation Centre to a new district in London. Needs support and local contacts in settling into her new home.'

'Mother of prisoner upset by parole refusal—needing support.'

'Prisoner requests a visitor for his parents aged seventy-eight and eighty-seven.'

Introducing the Voluntary Associates

In Chapter 9 mention was made of the need to prepare both parties before introduction. Practice varied as it did also in the means by which the voluntary associate was introduced to the client. In the case of a serving prisoner the first meeting was usually arranged by the welfare officer or the liaison probation officer who would often be present to make the introduction. This arrangement has sometimes been criticized on the grounds that it linked the voluntary associate with 'officialdom', but it may equally well be argued that it is helpful and fair for the client to know the reality of this relationship from the outset.

Occasionally, the initial meeting was arranged by the welfare officer, or the liaison probation officer, giving the client the voluntary associate's address and suggesting that the client might send him a visiting order. This arrangement was attractive in that it required initiative by the client by means of one of his few privileges, and it helped to make the relationship a personal transaction between the two parties from the outset. However, it made a heavy demand upon the client in having to write a covering letter to a stranger.

Where the client was in the outside community at the time of the first meeting the probation officer frequently made the introduction at his office, but often encouraged the two of them to go off for a talk in a local café after a short while. Again this made clear the voluntary associate's link with the probation officer.

The possibility of client and voluntary associate arranging an initial meeting on their own at such a café or on a street corner was too hazardous and created undue anxiety with which the client might well not be able to cope. The probation office offered a more familiar and more reassuring setting in the first instance.

Where the client was a wife then the initial contact was usually made by the voluntary associate visiting the home, but this arrangement was inappropriate for the single clients living in hostels or lodgings. The possibility of an initial meeting in the voluntary associate's home again raised problems and those who were willing to invite the client home generally felt that they needed several meetings to get to know him before introducing their family.

Contact during Sentence

The length of time between the initial contact with a prisoner and his date of discharge ranged from a few days to 4 years (see Table 18). Generally the referrals seemed to be late in the sentence, reflecting the point at which after-care plans are still made in many cases, but it must be remembered that many sentences are short. For borstal boys considerable progress was made in establishing earlier contact. (No figures can be given as the nature of the indeterminate sentence makes it difficult to estimate the date of release for those cases still under sentence.)

TABLE 18

Length of Contact Between Prisoners and Voluntary Associates Prior to Discharge

	%
Up to 1 month	23·2
Over 1 up to 3 months	12·8
Over 3 up to 6 months	19·2
Over 6 up to 9 months	14·1
Over 9 up to 12 months	6·4
Over 12 months	20·5
Not known	3·8
Total	100·0

N=78

Meetings between prisoners and voluntary associates were usually arranged by the former sending out his visiting order. If this was used regularly for a relative or friend then a special visiting order was often arranged with the co-operation of the governor and welfare officer. Either way the voluntary associate visited on much the same basis as a relative or friend. While this sometimes involved waiting and inconvenience it clearly established the ordinary nature of the visit and seemed preferable to privileged arrangements made through the welfare officer.

The basis of visits by the voluntary associate differed from that for a prison visitor. The former used the ordinary visiting rooms, had no special treatment, and visited just the one prisoner; the latter had a key and access to the cells, seeing a number of prisoners, a list usually having been prepared by the chaplain. Thus the prison visitor was more closely identified with the prison than the voluntary associate. Similarly, as we have noted, the prison visitor was frequently involved only during sentence, whereas the voluntary associate's visits were essentially preparatory for after-care.

The difficulties of building up a relationship in the austere setting of a prison, with a lack of external stimulus, must not be underestimated. Patiently over many visits, interspersed with letters if the visits were infrequent, a relationship of trust could develop so that the inmate began to feel that there was at least one person outside who cared and was willing to try to help him.

Contact after Discharge

During sentence the visits by the voluntary associate could follow a predictable timetable dependent upon his own availability and the visiting regulations. Once the prisoner was discharged, contact inevitably became less predictable. Similarly, the ex-prisoner often seemed very different. Thus the period immediately following discharge was frequently one of strain in the relationship and sometimes contact was lost at that stage.

Some voluntary associates met their clients at the prison gate, or on their arrival in London. Others arranged to meet on the first evening after discharge. Sometimes practical assistance in finding work or accommodation was a tangible expression of the voluntary associate's concern though often he was encouraged by the probation officer to help the client to help himself.

After a long period of isolation the need to cope with the rush of city life, to find one's way to all the various social agencies, and not to be disheartened by setbacks can be a major source of strain, sometimes resulting in an almost immediate breakdown. The voluntary associate (or sometimes a volunteer just for a day or so) could give support at this crucial stage.

No special provision was made for a meeting place. The temptation to provide an office or interviewing room where they could meet was resisted at the beginning of the project, on the grounds that it would have put the relationship on a formal footing, too similar to that between probation officer and client. Frequently meetings took place at cafes (or perhaps a public house if the client did not have an alcohol problem).

The lack of a meeting place sometimes created difficulties, especially for the women meeting male clients. It would have been easier if there had been some informal club room open several nights per week where they could meet in a reassuring setting, each finding support from the presence of other clients or voluntary associates.

Pressure was never put upon voluntary associates to invite their clients to their homes. Of the 121 who answered the questionnaire, 109 said that they had been put in touch with clients. Of these 22 (so far) had had contact during sentence only and a further 4 said that contact had been too brief to get round to inviting clients home. But 68 of the remainder said that they had done so, leaving only 15 who had not. In some instances it was difficult to invite them home, for example, when a wife was not keen for her husband to do so or for a single women. But many of those voluntary associates whose clients were still under sentence expressed their willingness to invite them home after their discharge.

Further indications of the voluntary associates' willingness to share their private lives with their clients was evident from the questionnaire. Fifty-one had introduced clients to members of their family and 43 to their personal friends. Only 25 had introduced clients to other voluntary associates, although several thought that this was a useful means of widening social contacts which they would hope to try in future. Similarly 25 had introduced clients to their 'church, club or other interest group'. Examples of such introductions were: voluntary associate and client jointly attending evening classes in art; a club for folk music which both attended; the voluntary associate invited the client to help him do odd jobs at a church and a community centre; a day out with an angling club; both attended working men's club etc. Not surprisingly in view of the personal beliefs of many of the voluntary associates, some invited their client to activities at their church, though this seems to have been done without pressure and after contact for some time.

Emotional Involvement
Where a relationship became well established a danger of over involvement easily resulted. Some emotional involvement was natural and necessary, especially for the more deprived or institutionalized clients. Dealing with only one or two clients the voluntary associate could afford to commit himself more emotionally than could the professional social worker.

Sometimes this led to the client acting out his problems within the relationship and to elements of transference from earlier relationships. One such situation showed how a strong mother-child relationship was established with an extremely immature young man. The intrusion of attitudes and feelings from his unhappy childhood created stress for the voluntary associate which would have taxed a professional worker, who might have been expected to recognize more readily the significance of his behaviour.

Voluntary associates learned to expect an uneven pattern of contact, but to be ready for a crisis at any time. One inadequate recidivist who had been out of touch with his voluntary associate for two months reappeared at his flat (where he had never been previously) at 11 p.m. in a drunken stupor and a severe state of physical exhaustion and emotional distress. While the young voluntary associate tried in vain to get the client readmitted to a mental hospital, from which he had recently discharged himself, his wife prepared a meal and a bed for the night. Not until noon on the following day was an admission arranged, after the voluntary associate had taken time off work.

Similar incidents could be recounted. They demonstrate the stresses under which the voluntary associates were placed from time to time, though it would be easy to overstate and to overdramatize. Even so the willingness to be available in a crisis and to put oneself out were vitally necessary qualities.

There was also the need to be willing to tolerate aggressive behaviour, for example, the alcoholic who rang his voluntary associate in a drunken state and in abusive terms said that he did not want to see him again. In more sober mood the hesitant efforts of the voluntary associate to resume contact were welcomed and regular meetings have continued for a further 2½ years so far.

But many clients were more passive and the relationships seemed rather routine. Sometimes inexperienced voluntary associates became concerned that they were not doing enough and needed reassurance to the effect that it was what they were *being* that perhaps mattered more. Incidents of manipulation or threatening behaviour were far less frequent than some might fear.

Work with Families
Work done by the voluntary associates with families tended to differ from that with individual clients. One or two voluntary associates were asked to make initial visits to wives when a request was received by the probation officer from the prison. Sometimes this involved just one visit to check that all was well, or some immediate help might be needed. At other times a more complex situation was discovered which the voluntary associate reported back to the probation officer. This could be regarded as involving the former in making a diagnosis of the family situation, but in practice it was much more a matter of gathering information so that the officer could then make an assessment indirectly.

Voluntary associates were also asked to give regular supportive visits to the wife and children in cases which had previously been visited by the probation officer. Sometimes this proved to be a means of making contact with the husband via the family. Then, as we have noted, either one or two voluntary associates could try to help the total family. This seemed to be a method that merited extension.

Contact with the Probation Officer

One hundred and fifty-nine of the clients were also in touch with probation officers (57 were not, 21 not known). This necessitated careful planning by the probation officer and the voluntary associate in each case so that they were clear as to their respective roles. A good understanding was needed to guard against a client trying to play one off against the other. Where a voluntary associate was in touch with a statutory after-care case or a probationer the maintenance of a relationship with the probation officer was essential, but triangular situations were not limited to these cases.

Reconvictions

Any systematic attempt to follow-up the clients to study reconvictions could be done only after a set period of time. It would in any case be extremely complicated to draw any conclusions from such a heterogeneous population (even if the non-offenders were excluded). In dealing with offenders, many of whom had long criminal records, frequent reconvictions were to be expected. On 49 occasions further offences were recorded after contact was established with the voluntary associate, in 5 cases there were 2 convictions during that time and in one, 3 convictions. These figures suggest that follow-up after, say, 2 years would reveal a high rate of recidivism.

The voluntary associates were taught to be prepared for further offences and not to give up as a result. Retaining close contact with the client at such a time of crisis, it was suggested, was a way of identifying with him and might strengthen the relationship for the future. Even when a client returned to prison the voluntary associate was encouraged to carry on.

When a client had to reappear in court it was natural that he should often want his voluntary associate to attend and perhaps 'speak on his behalf'. Most of the voluntary associates were, despite some apprehension about giving evidence, ready to do so, and to take time off work to attend court. This was encouraged by the probation officers and by the director. However, certain hazards had to be guarded against. Firstly, it was important that the voluntary associate should not be regarded by the court as someone qualified to express a professional opinion upon the defendant's conduct or likely response, if allowed to retain his liberty. Secondly, the voluntary associate could over-identify with the defendant, or sometimes be manipulated by him. However, many magistrates welcomed their comments and their interest which may have affected the courts decisions in some cases. Despite the occasional difficulties of voluntary associates who were inexperienced in the customs of the courts, there can be no questioning of the defendant's right to call his voluntary associate as a witness to his character, nor undervaluing of the probable psychological significance of standing by him at a time of crisis. Voluntary associates were encouraged to contact the probation officer on duty if a court appearance arose at short notice, so that they could be advised as to procedure in the court, and the clerk could be informed of the voluntary associate's status and interest in the case. When longer notice was given, it was possible to contact the consultant or supervising probation officer first.

Duration of Contact
The length of contact between voluntary associate and client varied. Some relationships were never really established or consisted of only one short contact; others lasted for years and seemed to be almost permanent. Two of the first 4 clients referred to the project were still in touch with their voluntary associates after nearly 3 years. Many of the contacts were still continuing and it would be impossible to predict their duration. Details of terminated and on-going relationships are given in Table 19.

TABLE 19

Duration of contact between voluntary associate and client

	Terminated Cases %	On-going Cases %
Up to 1 month	40·4	13·2
Over 1 month up to 3 months	10·6	4·7
Over 3 months up to 6 months	22·4	19·4
Over 6 months up to 9 months	13·8	22·5
Over 9 months up to 12 months	7·4	11·6
Over 12 months up to 24 months	5·4	20·2
Over 24 months	-	8·5
Total	100·0	100·1
Incomplete information 14		
	N=94	N=129

For the terminated cases it will be noted that contact in half these cases had ceased within 3 months, but taking terminated and on-going cases together it seems likely that the eventual average length of contact, when this can be calculated, will be very much greater.

However, no conclusions can be drawn from this information. Some relationships were only expected to be for one or two contacts; in others a few months may have been all that was necessary. Certainly there were some early breakdowns in the relationship where the probation officer had hoped for long-term contact. Some voluntary associates experienced several of these 'failures', and sometimes became disheartened. However, it was clear that on-going relationships could be established and with greater experience by probation officers in selecting cases, matching and introducing cases the number of failures to get under way seems to have begun to decline. This may, however, be the effect of referring more probation or statutory after-care cases.

CHAPTER 11

SOME ILLUSTRATIONS

In this chapter five illustrations are given of work undertaken by voluntary associates during the project. Each account has been prepared by a probation officer sometimes with the help of notes provided by the voluntary associates. These cases have been chosen to illustrate points made in previous chapters. It is not suggested that they are representative of a full cross-section of the work done, nor has any attempt been made to select only 'success stories'.

The first case 'John' shows how the voluntary associate made contact before the client's discharge from prison, although earlier contact during the sentence might have been desirable. It also shows the partnership between voluntary associate and probation officer who almost seem interchangeable, the former playing a role which might be thought to need professional skill.

Unfortunately, due to ill health, the voluntary associate had to withdraw from the relationship. Clearly this was a source of disappointment to the client and demonstrates the need to stay with a person for a long period, even though it was not possible in this case.

JOHN, AGE 28

John was in the last stages of a two-year sentence. The probation officer who had known him for many years was leaving and wanted someone to take over. He suggested a voluntary associate might be able to give the necessary support. John welcomed the idea when the probation officer next visited the prison. John is a young man who has spent the greater part of his life in institutions. He was sent to approved school, detention centre and borstal and from the time he was licensed from the last, offence followed offence, usually with only a few weeks between each one. The offences were nearly all connected with motor vehicles. His periods of liberty between prison sentences were short and there was no sign of his making any effort to break away from this pattern of behaviour. He seemed to have no ability to control his behaviour when at liberty and settled easily into the routine of any institution in which he found himself.

Shortly before the two-year prison sentence already mentioned he had married and he seemed to have (for the first time) some feeling of the need to settle and take on responsibilities. His wife was a hard worker and prepared to help him. She corresponded with him and visited him regularly in prison and at the time when the voluntary associate was suggested to him the future appeared set fair and more hopeful than at any previous time.

The probation officer took the voluntary associate, Michael, to meet John at the prison and this was successful. Only two visits were possible prior to discharge but almost simultaneously with these the bright future suddenly changed and John's hopes were shattered when his wife declared her intention of breaking up the marriage. Michael offered all the help and support possible, meeting the wife and then seeing both John and his wife together and separately almost daily after his release. John was not able to accept this shattering of all his hopes and became aggressive and resentful towards Michael when he thought too much sympathy was being shown to his wife, but after one particularly violent verbal explosion he was able to telephone and apologize. The turbulent week or two ended in John attempting to escape from his unhappiness by taking an overdose of drugs and being admitted to hospital. Almost at the same time his wife was also admitted to hospital after a car accident. Michael visited them both and continued to try to help them reach some reasonable compromise but John could not accept his wife's rejection and was therefore not able to give any thought to work or other problems of rehabilitation. The wife remained adamant in her refusal to consider attempting to establish a home together.

The situation could not continue at this highly emotional pitch and it was almost inevitable that John committed further offences after only about six weeks' freedom as a result of which he received a further twenty-one months' imprisonment.

This is no success story but the way in which the voluntary associate was accepted by John and his wife and the help he gave, certainly was invaluable to the couple at the time and the experience of the relationship has laid the foundations for work with John throughout his present sentence and one hopes for the future. Unfortunately Michael was not able to continue his contact for long after the start of John's present term of imprisonment because of ill health, but there is now a close relationship with the probation officer and the relationship with Michael seemed to pave the way for this. Letters from John frequently ask after Michael and kind messages are sent to him and indicating the warm regard which John has for someone who came from outside his own social circle, was not an official, but was certainly felt to be a helping friend.

PETER, AGE 21

Peter is an ex-borstal boy from an unhappy and unstable home, and with marked signs of psychological disturbance. His initial introduction to a voluntary associate was when she offered accommodation for home leave. From then onwards a lasting relationship was established and she and her husband became something of a substitute for his own family.

He is an intelligent young man, very concerned and angry because he did not use the educational opportunities given to him. He is the fourth of a family of eight children. Four of them attended grammar school as did Peter. Three elder brothers and one sister are now married, one of the brothers has served five years' imprisonment for robbery with violence. Peter's last offence also involved violence, when he and two others attacked a shop keeper and stole the contents of his till.

Peter's mother lives in Manchester and has in spasms been in contact with her family, who have all moved away from her immediate vicinity. He describes his mother as dominant and old-fashioned, almost victorian. His father died when Peter was twelve. Peter remembers him as a violent and aggressive drinker, who spent long periods away from home and who, on the occasions when he returned for a short period, created disharmony and at times terrified the family with his violence. Peter rebelled against his position very early in life by truanting and running away from home for short periods. At the age of 14 he was before the Court for failure to attend school. This set a pattern he has followed ever since through approved school and later borstal. He has had intense feelings of guilt and worthlessness and although he knows he has the intelligence to make a good constructive life and career, he has been self-destructive whenever his position has appeared to have improved. He rationalizes this attitude by constantly linking himself with his aggressive father and his elder brother who served the long prison sentence. To quote Peter, 'I said to someone once who was my friend, it is funny but eventually you will come to hate me because eventually I will make you hate me, and when he did hate me I took it that it was his fault.'

At the time when Peter was due for home leave shortly prior to his discharge to London as homeless, a member of Teamwork Associates, a Mrs White, agreed to provide him with accommodation and befriend him for the five-day period. She and her husband, a professional man, lived with their small daughter in an outer London suburb in unpretentious surroundings.

During the home leave period Peter was treated as one of the family, although he was rather non-plussed by this acceptance. 'What is in it for them—they cannot really like me?' He spent hours talking over his mixed feelings, hopes and ambitions, and Mrs White and her husband were good listeners, well able to contribute to the discussion at all levels when this was considered helpful. This proved to be a major factor in their later relationship with Peter who obviously needed to talk to somebody with a greater intellectual sense than he had himself. It also provided him with incentive to improve his own standards. At that time Peter had great difficulty in relating to Mr White. This was chiefly because he had no standards to judge him by other than those set by his father and brothers, prison officers, policemen or probation officers. This 'comparative judgement' has given Peter many hours of serious thought and has eventually led to lengthy discussions about his feelings.

At first even the accepted courtesies of—please, thank you, after you etc.—were embarrassing to him as he had considered them non-essentials and a sign of weakness. He also could not understand when or how he should use them. This proved to be the case with many of the everyday courtesies that go to the smooth running of a normal household. At times he became quite bewildered by his inability to understand this. Nonetheless he had developed a strong affection for the family, spending considerable periods amusing Mrs White's small daughter and even liking the family dog.

On return to borstal from home leave he wrote to Mrs White at length and also sent her poems he had written during his sentence. Like many persons who spend long periods in isolation, Peter spent hours writing poetry and short stories of a very deep and complex nature.

On release from borstal, he was found lodgings (bed-sitter) by me (the probation officer) and went to the job at a local bakery arranged during home leave. During his first few weeks he visited the Whites two or three times a week and on most other days he telephoned them at least once. He made it quite clear to me from the start that they were

his friends, but I was an official paid to supervise him. He could understand my involvement, but certainly could not at that time understand
theirs. He made it very obvious on occasions that this was his view of the
position and although Mrs White and I had many discussions on Peter's
progress at regular intervals, and were always quite open about this to
him, on most occasions Peter preferred 'not to know' or if he acknowledged that he did know he became very angry and jealous about it
being a three-way link.

After this early period, Peter decided to spread his wings, and as he
put it, prove he could do without 'us'. He gave up his job and his lodgings ('The thing that depresses me most is that I do not like living in a
room where my bed is'—an unwitting reference to his time spent in
cells), associated with drug addicts and other down and outs ('They are
much worse than I am, I can help them because I understand them').
Also during this period he went back to his home town for a weekend.
He later said that he had done so to confirm that his feelings for his
mother and the rest of his family were completely dead. During this
time he reported to me regularly, but our discussion was very formal.
I knew, however, that he had discussed his recent experimental activities with Mr and Mrs White and I was anxious not to interrupt this
dialogue. Much to the surprise of both Peter and Mrs White, most of
these discussions were on a man-to-man basis with her husband, with
whom Peter now related far better.

Shortly after this he became over-confident and with no warning
whatsoever he disappeared and nothing was heard of him for several
weeks. This led to much soul searching by Mrs White who found it
difficult to believe that Peter's disappearance was not due to some
omission on her part. She continued to feel this way in spite of my
constant reassurances that his disappearance was to be expected at this
time. When he did make contact with me by letter from a farm in
Yorkshire I had the greatest difficulty in dissuading her from sending
him a 'come back all is forgiven' plea. I knew that Peter's links with
her were sound, although he must work this out for himself. He
eventually moved on to visit his brother (just released from prison). He
again made contact with me from there, but did not contact Mrs White.
It was quite clear that he knew he must contact me as his supervising
officer, but he did not think he was worthy of contacting Mrs White at
that time or deserving of a reply. Some months later, however, he
arrived in London 'unexpectedly' and said he was just passing through.
Everything in Manchester was very good and he had a good job work-

ing at the same factory as his brother in the area, and he was staying with his brother and family. He called on Mrs White who was obviously delighted to see him again. He readily accepted her invitation to stay there for the weekend. He was amazed by this, but very pleased. After the weekend he returned to Manchester but a month later came back to London. He admitted that his stay in Manchester had really been disastrous. He had been frightened by the prospect of ending up as his brother had done and this had placed considerable pressure upon him. It had taken all his courage to break away from this and he admitted that his earlier visit to London had been made specifically to see whether he would once more be welcomed.

He was found accommodation and was accepted back at his old job. He soon returned to his former routine, visiting Mrs White and her family regularly. He also formed a friendship with some of Mrs White's neighbours and when one of these was in some difficulty he was quite sympathetic and helpful, something he could not have done spontaneously a few months previously. He was also slowly learning not to be suspicious of other people's actions quite so frequently. He was encouraged by Mrs White to renew his interest in his education, and as a result arrangements are in hand for Peter to commence part-time study for 'A' levels in English Language and English Literature in September. Here we have a satisfactory arrangement as Mrs White has supplied the incentive and given him the facilities for private study while I am providing the necessary help with books, stationery etc. for the more practical purposes.

At the moment there is no happy ending to this story as Peter is still very disturbed. During the past few months he has had several jobs and lost them. He has also lost accommodation. Most of this has happened not because of his inability to cope physically, or to do the job, but because of his own self-destructive impulses. He has at times spent long periods at Mrs White's, sometimes days on end, and recently she became quite apprehensive because she was concerned for her husband. Although he had said nothing he was suspected not to be too pleased at this constant intrusion on their privacy at increasingly frequent intervals. At this time she discussed the position with Peter as I did. It was only with great difficulty that he could understand what she or I meant by this, and on my advice she discussed this at greater length with her husband. It is only fair that she was not prepared to have her home life disrupted to such an extent, but Peter appeared to be totally committed to them and was at that time very much in need of such attention. When she discussed the matter with her husband, however, he said that he considered that it was very worth while. He had shown a keen personal interest in Peter and had decided that they should continue to do everything they could to help. In fact, at this stage Mr White was more the leading light in the arrangement than Mrs White. After this dangerous period had passed, Peter continued to see them very frequently and still stayed with them at times. He has now found a flat in that area and has also taken work there.

He continues to make extra friends and, while his future remains uncertain, he seems to be making slow, painful, but steady progress towards maturity and a better-balanced and more realistic view of himself and other people. He has also learned, by practical example, that life means giving as well as taking if it is to be lived to the full.

In my view, without the warmth and friendly simplicities and homeliness of Mrs White and her family, Peter would now be back inside, this time in prison.

ARTHUR, AGE 65

Arthur is an older man who might have been thought to be at a stage where little could be done to help him. Certainly the probation officer set low expectations in introducing a voluntary associate and the selection of a young single woman from a middle-class background for an 'old lag' may seem strange (but she was the only person available at the time). In fact her success in introducing him into her church, as well as in providing a personal relationship with him which is of some meaning to him, seems remarkable.

He is a widower. He has over 20 previous convictions mostly for petty larceny and false pretences, dating back to 1920. He has a long history of imprisonment including 8 years' preventive detention.

During recent years he has led a solitary life living in Salvation Army hostels and often finding it difficult to get work. I met him first two years ago when he was given a conditional discharge in court and he stated he would like to keep in contact with me on a voluntary basis. At that time he was a rather pathetic institutionalized man with no friends.

Initially he was out for what he could get. It transpired that he was simultaneously attending two probation offices asking for help and telling contradictory stories to the probation officers. He stayed at a Salvation Army Hostel, signed on regularly and was on the special list for older men, tried hard to find employment but failed to do so because of his record and his age. He reported very regularly—weekly, or at least fortnightly—and the interviews were strained and superficial, usually he talked about work or accommodation or his days in prison or his former career in the army, and always asked for his fares.

I felt strongly that here was a man who had the will to change, but could not find a facilitating environment for doing so. Furthermore, it was clear that he needed friendship and above all time—a scarce commodity for me to offer.

He eagerly accepted my propostion for a voluntary associate and when there was some delay in finding him one he became quite anxious. I had no strong views about what type of voluntary associate he should have and thought he could build a relationship with anyone prepared to give time and interest. Since that date Arthur has met Miss Webster regularly. She is a qualified nurse, a keen churchgoer, with a lively mind and a love of travel. Initially I wondered how it would work out— a young unmarried woman and an old lag in his sixties.

From the start Arthur was enthusiastic and it became immediately clear after having seen him regularly for six months that this relationship was able to impart to him something I had not been able to give— that he was acceptable to an ordinary member of the community, that he could meet informally in a café and talk to someone with no involvement in the penal services.

Initially he was suspicious. Yes, he liked Miss Webster but what was his relationship really about. This was the unspoken question. I learnt from her that in these early stages Arthur never talked about his days in prison.

Later he went to Brighton hoping for work. He stole £1 from a house at which he was making enquiries from a Salvation Army representative, and for this was placed on probation for two years. He clearly felt very ashamed of this offence and would not discuss it with me or Miss Webster. On arrival in London he made contact again with her and asked her for money.

Having found that both she and I were able to accept his having committed an offence without rejecting him there was a marked change in his behaviour. He had always been a man who found it difficult to give, but now slowly he started to show signs of wanting to help. This is a process which has continued since then and has shown in numerous ways, helping Miss Webster look for a car, taking her to various shows and exhibitions, doing odd jobs for other people.

Through her he was introduced to a club at her church. He attended this informal group every Thursday with her and through it became involved in a wider social group and church activities. At this stage he was still extremely dependent on both myself and Miss Webster.

He was then offered a job at the church as a part-time cleaner and quickly showed himself a hard and responsible worker. Shortly afterwards he was taken on full time. This gave him new life. Although still meeting Miss Webster regularly he became involved now with the life of the church and this gave him a real sense of purpose.

He spent Christmas with Miss Webster and her family and thoroughly enjoyed this. All the time he was increasingly showing his new-found pleasure in giving: sending Christmas cards, buying cups of tea, offering advice and was clearly beginning to feel a worthwhile citizen once again.

I moved house after Christmas and he offered to help decorate our new flat, and in fact came every weekend for about two months. Round about St Valentine's Day he was showing signs of having romantic feelings towards Miss Webster and also was having to get used to the idea of sharing me with my wife. For some weeks there were signs of unrest and dissatisfaction, but he seems to have resolved these and is able to accept that both myself and Miss Webster can only offer him limited time. She leads a busy life and Arthur takes great pride in her and talks in a fatherly way to me about her.

Without analysing too much one can state that through Miss Webster Arthur has been able to shift his identification with either a prison or hostel group to that of the church group. Had the relationship between him and Miss Webster remained on an exclusively one-to-one basis I think the age difference could have created difficulties. But now the relationship is firmly set within the wider social group and this encourages him to develop his own self-confidence, rather than to remain entirely dependent upon her. It is possible that she may be leaving London and I think that Arthur could now tolerate this as he has made sufficient links with a community through his work at the church. However, there is no doubt that these links would never have been made had he not been able to trust and have confidence in his voluntary associate in the early stages of readjustment.

FRED, AGE 50

Fred was an 'inadequate' and again someone for whom little seemed possible. The voluntary associate had to be helped to accept Fred's inability to make appreciable progress, yet to give him consistent support and encouragement and to try to prevent deterioration in his conduct. It is a good example of different but complementary roles by voluntary associate and probation officer. The case has been written up by a senior probation officer who was not directly involved—hence the references to the probation officer in the third person.

Fred was on probation for stealing and forging prescription forms in order to obtain barbiturate drugs. His probation began with a period in a mental hospital to attempt to resolve his drug dependency and after six months in hospital he was discharged to live with his elderly mother in her local authority flat. (He is separated from his wife and children who live elsewhere.)

In early 1968 after he had been home a year the probation officer recorded that: 'Fred induces in me an increasing feeling of helplessness. At one stage he reported regularly but now even his reporting has become erratic and I suspect that this is because I have put pressure on him to progress and that my disappointment at his failure to do so has conveyed itself to him. He tries to say the things that he believes will please me but never in fact *does* them; even the most trivial tasks seem beyond him; he does not work, scarcely moves from his mother's flat, has no social contacts and is becoming more and more like a vegetable. I fear that to increase the pressure on him to improve his position may force him further away from me and leave him without any social support and thus risk his return to drug dependency.'

This was the point at which it was decided to offer Fred the friendship of a voluntary associate. The first time the topic was introduced the probation officer talked with Fred about leisure and his admitted feelings of boredom. It was suggested that the probation officer 'knew a man who had offered to try to help people who had been in trouble by making friends and sharing interest'. It was very tentatively put and Fred rejected it saying he had a number of friends already. However, he went on to talk about the pleasures of watching football and said he hadn't been for years. . . .

Next time Fred came he raised the question of the voluntary associate and thought it might be nice to have someone to share outings with or who would help him in his search for work. He said timidly that he would like the associate to make contact with him at his own home first.

On his next visit Fred asked point blank whether any arrangement had been made for the voluntary associate to contact him. It was suggested that perhaps Fred could expedite this by telephoning him and later the same day the associate was given a more comprehensive picture of Fred.

Mr Williams was selected as the voluntary associate because he was a gentle but competent man who would not render Fred any more inadequate, but would provide support and reassurance and allow the probation officer to see whether increasing the pressure to find work was profitable.

Mr Williams wrote to Fred suggesting that Fred telephone him and as a result of the phone call a meeting was arranged on neutral ground (a Wimpy bar).

Thus began a regular contact, usually weekly. Mr Williams was soon welcomed into Fred's home where his elderly mother seemed to recognize her son's social isolation and his need for friends. Mr Williams gently began to extend Fred's social horizons; he was helped to cope with interviews at the employment exchange which for the first time referred him for a job (Fred didn't get it but he did attend the interview —another 'first'). With Mr Williams' help he joined the library and visited his son in a local children's home. Together, Fred and Mr Williams went on excursions to places of interest and the provision of an old radio by Mr Williams resulted in Fred beginning to interest himself in one or two practical tasks.

The probation officer's continued pressure on Fred to find employment produced an ineffectual truculence and a reluctance to report, but Mr Williams continued his regular contact and by liaison between him and the probation officer it was possible to ensure that Fred did not deteriorate or revert to drug-taking.

Mr Williams accompanied Fred for interviews to a number of jobs but his long period of unemployment plus his own diffidence militated against him and it seems likely that he was secretly relieved not to have to cope with starting a job. Nonetheless, Fred was now trying to undertake small tasks for himself and sometimes became quite pathetically boastful about some small enterprise or excursion.

The probation officer has now decided that to press Fred further about finding employment is unlikely to be productive but at least the attempt has been made without any deterioration in his behaviour.

Mr Williams continues his friendship, continually trying to widen Fred's horizons, always ready to help him make another attempt at finding work. He continues to visit the home and to provide small measures of practical help. (At present discussion is going on about whether the provision of an old motor-cycle would enable Fred to become more mobile and give him opportunities to gain confidence and add to his interests.)

Fred seems better in health than at any time since he has been on probation and he certainly copes a little better with simple routine matters. The only three 'props' Fred has at present are his mother, his probation officer and his voluntary associate. His mother's health is beginning to weaken (she is well into her eighties) and Fred's probation ends this year. His need for a voluntary associate is greater than ever if he is not to deteriorate.

WESLEY, AGE 24

The last illustration, Wesley, shows how two married couples and their families were all involved in giving support to a young man separated from his wife. It also shows how they and the probation officer together could give him a measure of interest which none of them could have given alone. A client with a profound sense of unworthiness was able to find some status through his relationships with these people. Contact terminated after some nine months when he left London and whether the help given will have any lasting effects remains to be seen.

This young man first became known to me when he was placed on probation five years ago. The offence was unlawful possession of firearms and it was a very unusual course for the court to take in view of the fact that he had some eighteen previous convictions. He had been remanded in custody for a probation officer's report and when I saw him in prison (this was the first time I had ever met him) we straight away seemed to get into a good relationship and in fact had a lengthy discussion there and then. The result was that because I felt I could work with him I recommended probation, although I never really expected that the court would agree.

Contrary to what sometimes happens in such cases Wesley continued to see me with regularity and our relationship began to develop. At that time he was a young man who was very conscious of his half-caste background, his father having been a West Indian. He was earning good money as a semi-skilled labourer but, unfortunately, this was not enough to give him the status which he felt he required and to supply him with all the necessary worldly goods to make him equal to his pure white contemporaries. The result was that he was very soon in trouble, a case of armed robbery together with three others, and was finally committed to five years' imprisonment.

After his committal I visited his wife and their, then, two children in their one-roomed flat. I endeavoured to persuade her to rejoin her parents who at that time were living in another part of the country. She resisted my efforts and their requests to return and it soon became obvious that she regarded her husband's committal to prison as giving her a new-found freedom, for she began to associate with various men and in fact became extremely promiscuous, her reputation being known throughout the neighbourhood. At first she said this was only a temporary thing and that she would return to her husband when he was released, but her way of living soon dulled any finer feelings within her and after a year or so she decided that she did not want to have any more to do with Wesley. During the four and a half years that her husband was away she produced two children, both by different men, and was pregnant by yet another man at the time of his release.

For the majority of his sentence Wesley was in only one prison and formed a very good relationship with the welfare officer there. I also wrote to him almost every week that he was away and he replied equally frequently. His letters were introspective and this long sentence gave him opportunities to think about life in a way which he had never bothered to do before. He also took various classes offered by the prison in English etc. and improved himself academically. It was, of course, a great blow to him when he had to face up to the fact that his wife was being unfaithful to him and that she had expressed the wish not to live with him upon his release, but somehow he managed to do this although there was a period of great depression and also some violence towards the prison staff at this time.

When I was considering Wesley's release I realized that he was going to need an enormous amount of support, he had no home, no wife, no job and no money either. Everything in fact tended to underline his former feelings of inferiority centred around his colour. The only positive factor in this situation was the good relationship which I had with him.

On the day of his release I met him at Euston Station together with a friend of mine who agreed to put him up for a short while. We had a meal together and made the usual applications to the Ministry of Social Security and the Labour Exchange. I realized that even on his first evening Wesley was going to be at a loose end and so I casually suggested that he might like to come with me to meet some friends of mine. These were, in fact, Mrs Jenkins, a voluntary associate and her husband. I did not mention to him at the time their semi-official connection with me, I was not in any way creating a false situation because I do genuinely regard them as my friends and indeed have endeavoured to enter into a bond of friendship with all the voluntary associates with whom I am connected. I do this because I feel that the client can accept them better this way, almost as though they are an extension of myself. Wesley's response to the Jenkins was somewhat suspicious at first. Mr Jenkins wears a beard and for a few days Wesley was convinced that he was a psychiatrist and was endeavouring to 'bend his mind in some way'. Their response to him, however, was warm and open-hearted. He was given an open invitation to visit their home and after some initial reluctance availed himself of this opportunity once or twice a week. His fears concerning Mr Jenkins were soon dispelled.

At this time Wesley was working in a rather menial job. The money was not very good but it was all he could obtain with his rather poor record. He needed extra money wherever it could be found, he had been trained as a barber in prison and the Jenkins asked him to cut their children's hair which he did very well. This gave me the opportunity to introduce him to another couple who are voluntary associates, Mr and Mrs Peters. They had two boys and he cut these boys' hair and in this way came to know the Peters and had an open invitation to visit them, an invitation which he availed himself of from time to time.

At one point a crisis arose because he lost his job through poor time-keeping. (He found it very difficult to get up in time for the odd hours that he was required to do on shift work). He came to my office in a very despondent state, in fact burst into tears. I immediately contacted Mrs Jenkins who came down to the office within a few minutes. She is a warm-hearted person and was able to put her arms around Wesley and comfort him. It was obvious that this meant a lot to him and in this way this particular crisis was averted.

Right from the moment he was released Wesley had decided that he wanted to employ his spare time in the most profitable manner and in fact signed himself for evening classes in psychology and short-story writing. The Jenkins interested themselves in these matters too and had many discussions with Wesley on these subjects, often lasting late into the evening. Mr Jenkins is a member of a discussion group and he took Wesley along with him on some Saturday evenings. It soon became known there that Wesley was an ex-prisoner and he was often given an opportunity to speak about his feelings about prison. This, I suppose, gave him some sort of status.

The Peters were rather different in their approach from the Jenkins. They are Christian people and in some respects appear rather strict. Nevertheless they too, like the Jenkins, are a very warm and loving couple and this soon enabled Wesley to accept them despite what he probably felt at the beginning was a certain austereness about their beliefs. He has, in fact, attended their church on several occasions and had useful and helpful discussions both with them and the pastor there. I think he sees their well regulated and well organized family life as something he would like to have for himself.

It would be pleasant to be able to finish this story on a happy note, but unfortunately tragedy struck and the eldest of Wesley's two small boys was quite recently killed in a road accident. He was only six years old and he and his brother had been frequent visitors at their father's flat. He used to invite them up there almost every weekend. On hearing the news Wesley came immediately to my office, but unfortunately I was not available and it is interesting that he then turned to the Jenkins for support. Both they and the Peters have helped him enormously during this very difficult time. The Peters and other friends whom he had made through his contact with them attended the child's funeral and comforted him there. Now Wesley has the sole care of his younger son. It has not been possible for him to remain in London so he has returned to live with his parents in Birmingham. I know, however, that he will keep in contact with all of us as he has promised to do for I believe he has made real and lasting friendships which at the moment have enabled him to survive more than one serious crisis, something which I am sure he would not have been able to do without turning to crime some years ago.

As an after thought and thinking over what I have said, it seems perhaps that Wesley was on the receiving end of everything all the time. This was not so, however, and indeed one would not have felt that there would have been any measure of success if it were. It is true that both the Jenkins and the Peters made the first advances to him, inviting him into their homes and giving him meals, but sometime before he left London he had invited both them and myself on two or three occasions to dinner at his flat. He is quite a good cook and was proud to be able to give us an excellent meal each time. I feel that Wesley has been helped especially because his voluntary associates were able to accept him despite the fact that he had had so many convictions, some of them for violence, that they were also able to give him 'room' to express himself despite the fact that some of the opinions that he voiced (at first, at any rate) were foreign and may have been distasteful to them. Lastly, and perhaps most important, they were willing and happy to receive things from him.

CHAPTER 12

SUPERVISION

If voluntary associates undertake work of the kind described in the last chapter a close working relationship with the probation officers is essential. Almost all the voluntary associates welcomed regular support and consultation. Occasionally a voluntary associate tended to become over-dependent or, alternatively, might fail to consult the probation officer for fear of being a nuisance or because he was thought to be too busy, but most recognized, in a mature way, their dependence upon the skill and experience of the probation officer.

In Chapter 5 we acknowledged the limited objectives which must be set for a brief preparation course. In the final session of each course great stress was put upon the need to learn from subsequent experience. But to have an experience is not necessarily to learn from it. For the voluntary associate learning from experience involved the readiness to accept that he as well as the client was likely to be changed through their relationship. If he was willing to put himself at risk in this way, then the relationship began to become more reciprocal and less patronizing. As we shall see in the next chapter, many of the voluntary associates recognized that they had been changed by their experience.

But the willingness to change depended upon a sense of security, which in turn was helped by the regular and consistent support of other voluntary associates and probation officers. In discussion with them there was the opportunity for self examination and to question established attitudes in a secure and safe setting. Thus a means of learning from experience was provided.

The second Reading Report[1] stressed the importance of regular contact with the probation officer:

'It is essential that information and guidance should be continuously available to him (the voluntary associate), and he should expect to learn year by year from his experience with offenders and his regular discussion with probation officer's.'

Responsibility and Accountability

Equally important is the need for the voluntary associate to account for his work. The 1965 Home Office Circular[2] said:

'While a volunteer may undertake substantial help in an individual case, the probation officer concerned must retain full responsibility. The volunteer's responsibility is to the probation officer concerned, with whom he will need to maintain close contact.'

The interpretation of 'full responsibility' is not easy. Clearly the voluntary associate has a responsible job to do and must frequently take decisions, particularly in helping clients at times of crisis, without the opportunity to consult the probation officer first. If, however, we take the circular to mean 'overall responsibility' this in no way diminishes the need for the voluntary associate to be accountable to the probation officer.

The experience of Teamwork Associates suggested that formal reporting back in writing was unworkable and often unhelpful. Voluntary associates were reluctant to make reports and there was a risk of making the contact with the probation officer too rigid. In practice, regular discussion between voluntary associate and probation officer was preferred by both.

Supervision

The meaning of the word 'supervision' is wider in social work practice than in everyday usage. Thus for the voluntary associate supervision did not simply mean overseeing his work; it also meant providing support and clarification. As in the preparation courses there were dangers here of inadvertently leading the voluntary associate into a quasi-professional role which might have detracted from his distinctive contribution.

Supervision was not equally acceptable to all voluntary associates. One, for example, said that he was glad to work 'with', but not 'under the supervision of', the probation officer. In any case, the supervision of a volunteer must differ somewhat from that of a paid employee, but most voluntary associates in practice, if not in name, entered into a relationship of supervisee with the probation officer as supervisor.

Methods of Supervision

In the early stages of the project the voluntary associates worked exclusively with the director. This helped him to gain some experience and some idea of the type of supervision needed. In any case, there were few probation officers sufficiently involved with the project to share the task at that stage. It was, however, a demanding and time-consuming job. As the project grew it was clear that the director could not hope to supervise more than perhaps 30 voluntary associates and even then it would deflect his energies from recruitment, training and the general development of the work. Thus the growth of the project beyond this size seemed to be possible only by providing far less supervision, or involving others as supervisors.

One way of doing the latter, tried by some other projects, was to invite the referring officer to undertake the full responsibility for supervision. But he was unlikely to have much experience of working with voluntary associates. If the original referral had been from a prison welfare officer, the chances of the voluntary associate establishing a strong link with a probation officer once the prisoner was discharged seemed remote. Arrangements of this sort seemed too haphazard, too fragmented and provided no means of intensive learning from experience for the supervisor as much as for the voluntary associate.

As explained in Chapter 2, it was decided that the formation of small groups or teams, each with a probation officer as 'consultant', offered a possible model which would be complementary to the supervision of the individual probation officer in many instances. It was also a model suggested by the Home Office Circular[3] and by the second Reading Report.[4]

The Teams

Experience seemed to show that a team with an optimum of 7 to 9 voluntary associates enabled them to use meetings profitably and engendered a supportive atmosphere. Some teams were smaller, especially in the early stages of starting in a borough and it was found that they lacked buoyancy. At the other extreme, some teams grew to be as large as 16 and 18 members which presented different problems. Members did not always have the opportunity to discuss their work during a session, nor the consultant the chance to check on how each member was getting along. Intimate discussion became more difficult, and absence from meetings less conspicuous and, therefore, more likely.

Most teams met monthly for an evening, usually at a probation office, but particular ones at a church, a rectory, a club for ex-prisoners, and members' homes. Some teams became more confident than others and more adventurous in their work. To some extent these traits reflected those of the consultant. Basically, however, the teams adopted similar working methods. Most meetings started with an opportunity for members to share with each other how things had been going since they last met. From this one or more problems might emerge which the team could then discuss more fully. Alternatively, if there were no pressing problems, a question of more general interest might emerge for discussion.

In one borough with 11 voluntary associates the pattern was different. Smaller groups of 3 or 4 members were assigned to work each with a probation officer, and the whole number only came together periodically for more general meetings, or to hear visiting speakers from local social services. One advantage of this arrangement was that several probation officers were fully involved which helped to generate interest and a willingness to refer cases to voluntary associates.

Like any other small groups, the morale of the teams changed over time and they experienced moods of elation and depression. Similarly the relationship with the probation officer varied from total dependence to, in one or two instances, periods when his leadership was questioned, but overall the experience seemed to be one of growth toward greater individual and group maturity. This was evident in an increasing ability to withstand disappointments and, especially, to support an individual member when he was facing crises or depressed by setbacks. At the same time members began to discover for themselves an identity as voluntary associates, a kind of composite image, built up from the sum total of their experience. This helped them to see themselves as distinct from the probation officers and reduced the risk of over-identification with their attitudes and work habits.

Some Problems

It will be evident from these comments that great stress was put on the local teams and they were regarded as the key point, not only in the relationship between voluntary associate and probation officer, but also in the project as a whole. However, several problems were experienced and not all of them were satisfactorily resolved.

In some teams the consultants were the sole source of referrals to the voluntary associates, but in the others most referrals came from colleagues locally and from prison welfare officers. In these instances, the consultant was unlikely to know the client and this made it much more difficult for him to make an accurate assessment of a situation described by the voluntary associate and to give appropriate advice. The situation was similar to that between a senior probation officer and a probation officer under his supervision, but with the difference that the latter could be expected to present a more detailed and more objective description and to play a more active part in working towards a solution of the problems presented. With a voluntary associate, particularly an inexperienced one, the consultant could be in some doubt as to the accuracy of a description given.

Where another probation officer was in touch with the client, or at least knew him, the consultant could confer with him, but there was a further problem to be resolved in these circumstances. What were the respective roles of the two probation officers *vis-à-vis* the voluntary associate? Inevitably practice varied. Some voluntary associates established an understanding with one probation officer with whom they worked closely over a number of clients. When this happened the voluntary associate tended to look for a more general opportunity to learn from experience in team sessions and to take particular problems to 'his own' probation officer. But where that probation officer was inexperienced in supervision, or failed to grasp the need for the voluntary associate to be supervised, the consultant often found himself having to take over this function. This was clearly unsatisfactory, but unavoidable until many more probation officers have experience of working with voluntary associates.

These problems were discussed fully by the consultants. Ideally, it was thought, the voluntary associate should be accountable to the probation officer who was in regular contact with the client and would therefore be the 'supervisor'. The 'consultant' would then be free, as his title implied, to be available in the background to advise and support both probation officer and voluntary associate as necessary, and to look after the continuing needs of the voluntary associate beyond the limits of a particular case.

Where no supervisor, in this sense, was involved, e.g. when an ex-prisoner was referred by a prison welfare officer before discharge, either a particular probation officer would have to be nominated to become the supervisor or, more probably, the consultant would, as at present, act in a dual capacity. Similarly he would continue to have a combined role where he referred one of his own clients to a voluntary associate. But experience suggests that a sharper distinction between his supervisory role, perhaps conducted individually, and his consultative role in the group setting, could obviate some of the difficulties experienced during the project. It could also relieve some of the pressures from over-burdened group discussions in which each member feels obliged to give an account of his case. However, it would tend to increase still further the demands upon probation officers' time whether the supervisor and the consultant were the same or two different people.

The voluntary associates' views as to the most valuable source of advice were requested in the questionnaire and their answers are included in Table 20.

TABLE 20

Voluntary Associates' Opinions as to the Most Valuable Source of Advice in their Work

	%
The individual probation officer who knows the client	53·7
The consultant probation officer alone even when he does not know the client	5·8
The team, including the consultant probation officer	25·6
Another voluntary associate	–
Other	1·7
Don't know	1·7
More than one answer given	4·1
No information	7·4
N=121	100·0

*These were two voluntary associates, one working closely with a psychiatrist and the other with a psychiatric social worker.

Individual contact with the probation officer concerned was valued more than that of the team. All (excluding the 'don't knows' and 'no information') selected an answer which included a probation officer.

Another problem which was of more immediate concern to some of the voluntary associates was whether the client would object to being talked about in the team. As members accepted the same standards of confidentiality as probation officers, the situation was analogous to discussion in a probation officers' case conference. But behind this problem lay the more difficult one of how the voluntary associate could be accountable to the probation officer, yet not appear to be a spy for him. Often clients grasped the nature of the relationship and did not raise any objections, and most voluntary associates sought neither to emphasize nor to deny their link with the probation officers.

A problem of quite a different order was how to introduce new voluntary associates into an established team. If the newcomer did not share a similar outlook to that of the team, it was feared by some consultants that this would cause difficulties. Despite their anxiety, this did not prove to be a serious problem in practice. It is in the nature of a small group that members tend to adopt a similar outlook and the newcomer was usually ready to learn from more experienced members. To avoid a team becoming too exclusive there was merit in introducing new members fairly frequently, and in reminding existing members that this was the normal practice.

It was also important to keep the team task-centred so that discussion of personal matters was seen to be relevant only insofar as it related to their voluntary associate work. In practice, all concerned seemed to recognize this and there was no cause to fear a shift into a therapeutic group situation.

Although a number of the consultants were interested in group methods, none had specialized training in group work. Those who were senior probation officers had, of course, experience in running staff groups which were not dissimilar, but there was no ready made method to adapt for the voluntary associate team. It had to be learned by trial and error. There is a need to establish some rationale for group work of this kind. It may be that experience in allied fields, for example, by Balint[5] with groups of general practitioners, could be applied, especially if expert leadership could be provided to help a group of consultants to examine their working methods more closely.

REFERENCES

1. Op. cit., par. 44.
2. Op. cit., par. 18.
3. Ibid., par. 19.
4. Op. cit., par. 45.
5. See R. Gosling and others, *The Use of Small Groups in Training*, Codicote Press 1967.

CHAPTER 13

———

SOME EFFECTS OF THE PROJECT

The Problem of Evaluation
At the beginning of this report it was stressed that systematic evaluation
had been precluded. Funds were not available to employ research staff,
nor had it seemed feasible to set up a controlled experiment. The need
to modify the project as it progressed to take account of circumstances
confirmed the assumption that a more rigidly planned project would
have been inappropriate. It is also arguable that any attempt to subject
the work of voluntary associates to such a rigorous evaluation would
have been premature. Time was needed for them and the probation
officers to gain some experience first.

It would, in any case, be unwise to attempt to evaluate the project
solely in terms of its effects upon the clients. In this chapter we shall
consider also effects upon the voluntary associates themselves. In the
long-run projects of the Teamwork Associates type may affect the community at large, and already some effects are evident upon the Probation and After-Care Service and, to a lesser extent, on the Prison
Service. It would, however, be an exaggeration to suggest that just
one pilot project had such effects, except of a marginal nature.

The Clients
Any attempt to evaluate the project in terms of effects on the clients
raises the problem of defining 'success'. For the purpose of official statistics, this is often taken to mean not being reconvicted during a stated
period after discharge from an institution, or during the currency of a
probation order. Even if these were to be taken as measures for those
offenders dealt with by the project, it could be misleading to attribute
any 'success' to the efforts of the voluntary associate, rather than to
those of the institutional staff, the probation officer or to extraneous in-
fluences. In any case without reliable prediction scores or controlled
experiments no comparison of expected and actual reconviction rates
could be made.

Nor is reconviction necessarily the most appropriate measure. Sometimes there has been a tendency to assess the voluntary associate's 'success' in terms of length of contact with the client. Certainly breakdown after one or two contacts when it had been hoped to establish a long-term relationship can be regarded as failure. But the length of a relationship is no measure of its quality, nor of its value to the client. Sometimes one or two contacts may be all that is needed, for example, in helping a client to find lodgings. At the other extreme a seemingly endless relationship may be a mark of the voluntary associate's own need to maintain the relationship, or of the client's failure to establish links in the community. There are wide variations in the optimum length of contact according to the needs of the client. Thus it seems to have little value as a measure of 'success'.

A third possible criterion for 'success' could be based upon the client's progress in establishing or re-establishing relationships in the community with parents, wife, girl-friend or his peers. Similarly stability in his place of residence and employment, and involvement in social activities might be measured. But again any progress or change thus measured cannot necessarily be attributed to the efforts of the voluntary associate.

During the preparation courses the voluntary associates were encouraged to set their sights low, to expect little progress, yet not to give up hope. Some attached more importance than others to seeing some change for the better, but the view expressed by Holden[1] with regard to the voluntary associates of the Blackfriars Scheme was probably true of them too:

'Most associates are not primarily interested in reducing crime, nor even in the moral reform of their clients. They are concerned to befriend someone whose life has, until now, been a misery to himself and to others, and to try to bring some happiness into his world by enabling him to form, perhaps for the first time, a stable relationship with someone whose motives, as far as he is concerned, are disinterested.'

The relief of suffering, or the restoration of personal dignity and worth, can be regarded as ends in themselves. The very act of offering help, whether accepted or rejected by the client, whether it helps him or not, can be seen as an expression of justice. In traditional retributive terms it may be argued that, as it was just to punish the offender so it is equally an expression of justice to offer him acceptance and help when he has paid the price for what he did wrong. Thus, the voluntary associate, as much as the judge or magistrate, can be seen as an agent of the community through whom it dispenses justice. At this level the voluntary associate's work has a moral value in absolute terms and independent of results, even if these could be measured.

In practice, evaluation becomes individualized and subjective. The referring probation officer or the voluntary associate himself may have certain expectations, and if these are fulfilled may feel that the latter was in some way instrumental in bringing about progress. For some clients such expectations may be total reintegration into the community and a final break with crime, but for another they may be simply that this time he may stay out of prison just for a few weeks, or maybe months, longer than last time. As in psychiatric practice, the revolving door principle often applies, where length of time outside the institution relative to that inside is a crude measure of progress or success. As we have noted, many of the probation officers were doubtful about the value of voluntary associates and resistant to any suggestion of referring clients to them. But those probation officers who were involved with voluntary associates, almost without exceptions, became enthusiastic about their contribution and were keen to explore ways of helping them to play a bigger part in the work. In practical terms this was the most crucial evaluation.

No systematic evaluation of professional social work, including probation work, has yet been conducted to establish its effectiveness, and research methods of the controlled experiment type raise substantial practical and ethical problems. In the absence of evaluative studies of professional work, it may be argued that it is premature to attempt to apply such methods in voluntary work, but in the long run they will be essential for both.

The Voluntary Associates

It may seem odd to attach much significance to the effects upon the voluntary associates. If, however, they are seen as the nucleus of a new generation of workers in the voluntary after-care field, and as means of modifying public opinion, then their capacity to learn from experience is clearly important.

It would be surprising if the voluntary associates had not been changed by their experiences. In their answers to the questionnaire 57 of them thought that their 'general outlook on life' had been affected and 78 that their 'attitude towards offenders' had been affected. The following were some of the comments made:

Effects on General Outlook on Life

'It has broadened my outlook considerably.'

'I think that I have become far more tolerant.'

'It has made me realize that help does not always need to be in concrete terms.'

'I am now slightly more cynical or realistic.'

'I no longer judge people on my own standards (not that I live up to them!) Seriously, I think understanding and tolerance are two things I am learning.'

'A difficult question to answer because I tend to throw away my worn-out attitudes like worn-out socks.'

Effects on Attitudes towards Offenders

'I look on them with more sympathy and understanding.'

'I find a benevolent attitude more difficult in practice than in theory.'

'It has made me less impatient and I think more understanding of their problems. At times I find myself on their side against authority.'

'My purpose was to "reform". I now feel that, of course that is a desirable objective, but that the relationship is a worthwhile end in itself regardless of "success".'

'I used to be frightened of prisons and their inmates. I don't mind going to prison a bit now.'

'It has shown me the necessity for accepting them as they are, and perhaps as they wish to remain.'

'I am less resentful when my house is broken into.'

An interesting future study might compare the attitudes of voluntary associates before and after their experience with one or more clients. In the meantime, the above comments tend to confirm the general impression that exposure to face-to-face contact with offenders helps to reduce prejudice and fear based upon ignorance.

The Community

This process of learning by the voluntary associates can be regarded as a modest contribution to educating the public. They in turn may be an educative influence upon their family, friends and workmates, so helping to create pockets of awareness and interest in the problems of offenders. The willingness of voluntary associates to introduce clients to their family or friends (p. 97) is encouraging in this respect. Of the 121 who completed the questionnaire no less than 119 said that their personal friends knew about their work as a voluntary associate (no information from 2 respondents). Not all these friends were sympathetic as the following comments showed, but at least there were signs that they were being called upon to re-examine some of their opinions.

'Most doubt the wisdom of such work—but most of my friends are hard-boiled!'
'They are very helpful—full of good ideas. The next step is to push them into action.'
'They keep telling me that I could do something for worthier people in need.'
'They think I am nuts.'
'Friends of my own age and leanings present no problems. My parents are another matter.'

How far the voluntary associates have contributed so far to a better informed or more tolerant body of opinion in the community is problematical. Most of them were more concerned to get on with the job. They did not particularly want to attract attention and were conscious of the need to respect the confidence of their clients. Fifteen of the voluntary associates had spoken to small meetings of churches or voluntary organizations. With greater experience others might well be able to take a more active part in giving talks to groups in their local community, but during the three years most requests for a speaker were met by the director in person. Towards the end of the project, probation officers began to ask for information to incorporate in the talks which they were asked to give.

These talks can be viewed as part of slow but persistent attempt to modify public opinion and to correct prejudice arising from ignorance or misleading sensational reporting of some crimes. At the same time a network of contacts was built up, with individuals and organizations that could be tapped in the future.

In the process of establishing these contacts and talking to leaders of organizations, it became painfully clear how ill-formed they were about the work of the Probation and After-Care Service. Those who had any knowledge of after-care were often unaware of the reorganization following the ACTO Report. Clearly there was a public relations job to be done which could not be undertaken adequately by the staff of a voluntary organization, however close its link with the statutory service.

One small project could not expect to make much impact upon public opinion, or contribute much to the process of community education. However, it became clear that a real opportunity existed which a well co-ordinated effort by statutory and voluntary services could tackle.

The Probation and After-Care Service

A major concern, throughout the project, was to help probation officers examine the case for involving voluntary associates, initially in relation to the new developments in after-care. At the same time, an attempt was made to overcome the crisis of confidence between the statutory service and the voluntary organizations. Within Inner London, the director talked to probation staff meetings and conferences and to trainee officers, but involvement in preparation courses for voluntary associates and selection panels perhaps did more to engender interest among officers.

The voluntary associates were, in effect, ambassadors for Teamwork Associates and for the wider voluntary movement in after-care. By their efforts on the job, probation officers began to take an active interest in working with them. A nucleus of perhaps 30 probation officers was established who were keenly committed to exploring ways in which voluntary associates could help. However, they were only about 10 per cent of the probation officers in Inner London and, even at the end of the project, many of the remainder had not had any contact with the project or with similar work under different auspices. Those with little or no involvement in after-care tended to see voluntary associates as beyond their immediate field of work.

Outside Inner London the director corresponded with, met, or addressed many probation officers interested in similar projects. These meetings were a valuable exchange of experience and ideas and it was possible to contribute to the planning of several other projects.

With other projects up and down the country, Teamwork Associates can perhaps claim to have contributed to changes of attitude and practice in the Probation and After-Care Service which is beginning to do more to mobilize the resources of the community.

The Prison Service

In view of its close ties with the Probation and After-Care Service, the project did not establish such strong links with the Prison Service as was achieved by some prison-based projects. The opportunity to make contact with prison staff was not developed. It can be argued that voluntary associates should avoid too much involvement with the institution if they hope to win the confidence of inmates, but the experience of the Youth Resettlement Project in gaining the active support of governors and their assistants suggested that this was of great value in establishing pre-release relationships with inmates.

Efforts to establish closer links with the staff of institutions must not be seen purely in terms of the preparation for after-care. They can also be a means of breaking down their isolation and helping them to feel less misunderstood by the outside public. Thus voluntary associates may have an effect upon the institution by bringing in something of the outside world for the staff as well as for the inmates.

The Object of a Pilot Project
The object of a pilot project is essentially exploratory. Part of its value lies in testing new ideas in practice so that others may capitalize on its achievements and try to avoid its shortcomings. Exploratory work of this sort, and attempts to record the experience gained, can be regarded as a necessary pre-requisite before embarking upon more rigorously conducted experiments incorporating evaluation by independent research workers.

REFERENCE
1. H. M. Holden, 'The Voluntary Associate Scheme', *British Journal of Criminology* Vol. 4 No. 4., April 1964.

CHAPTER 14

SOME IMPLICATIONS FOR FUTURE PROJECTS

Although the project described in the previous section had an immediate and practical purpose, its primary objective was to gain operational experience, to put to the test some of the proposals contained in official reports, and to feed back what was learned in the hope that it would prove to be of some value in planning future developments.

Needless to say, events did not stand still during the three years of the project. It has been a time of growing activity by probation officers in various parts of the country to involve volunteers. Except perhaps in its organizational structure, Teamwork Associates could make no claim to be unique. There is a pressing need to compare the experience gleaned from different projects in different types of area.

Any attempt to draw implications from the Teamwork Associates project must be made with caution for two reasons: first, conditions in Inner London present different problems and also different opportunities than in other parts of the country; second, the project was launched at a time when the redevelopment of after-care was still at an early stage and many of the circumstances which influenced decisions in planning the project no longer apply.

Recruitment
That Teamwork Associates experienced no special difficulty in finding voluntary associates of high calibre was encouraging. With a Greater London population of about 8 million to draw upon it might be claimed that a London based project had an advantage over those in the provinces, but discussion with probation officers running projects in provincial cities reveals adequate numbers of recruits. In all areas the response has been mainly from the middle class.

For centuries organized voluntary work has been the prerogative of the upper and middle classes. Long-standing traditions will not be changed overnight although there are signs that the range of social background is getting wider. The Aves Report[1] quoted a number of surveys of volunteers in the social services, all of which showed the dominant contribution of the middle class. But the Committee found some evidence to support the belief that 'willingness to help other people exists and is translated into action at all levels of society' though this was frequently of a more spontaneous and less organized kind in working-class communities.

It may well be that it has been a mistake in after-care to appeal for working-class support for organized voluntary service, rather than to recognize and mobilize the resources of good neighbourliness and comradeship on the factory floor in a much more informal and spontaneous way. Deciding how this could best be done calls for much imagination. There would, for example, be value in testing a method of recruitment tried in Holland where the prisoner is invited to name a person known to him and perhaps resident in his home neighbourhood, to be his 'voluntary associate'. This individual is then approached by the after-care agency and invited to help. He may, of course, be middle class, but frequently would be from a working-class background. (This, incidentally, constitutes a useful form of matching.)

If by means such as this a new kind of 'informal' voluntary associate can be introduced, there will be an opportunity to compare his effectiveness with that of the existing kind of 'formal' voluntary associate. No project has yet involved enough working-class voluntary associates to give a clear guide as to their distinctive contribution. There is a strong case for a pilot project, perhaps under the leadership of a probation officer with a trade union background, to explore ways of mobilizing help from trade unions, trades councils, working men's clubs and so on.

But to argue the case for such a project must not be taken to imply criticism of the present voluntary associates. The capacity to care, to understand, and to respond constructively to the needs of others is not destroyed by barriers of social class. Experience suggests that the social distance from the clients, or a measure of detachment, can frequently be an advantage and may be more acceptable to some clients. The need, therefore, may not be to recruit a different kind of voluntary associate but to widen the range of recruitment.

The decision of the Home Office[2] to encourage local recruitment rather than a 'national recruiting drive' would seem to have been wise. There can be little doubt that projects like Teamwork Associates would have benefited from any attempt to create a more receptive climate of opinion among the public. But unless there was a recognized need for voluntary associates throughout the country, and adequate machinery to use them and supervise them a national approach could do more harm than good. Instead there may be a case for local use of mass media, such as local radio, both for public education about offenders and for stimulating the recruitment of volunteers.

Training

Methods of preparation developed by Teamwork Associates may seem over formalized. In some areas training has been concurrent with practical experience, i.e. after the voluntary associate has been introduced to his first client. This is superficially attractive, enabling the voluntary associate to become involved quickly and offering experience as the basis for learning. A skilled tutor/supervisor may pick up much teaching material from the voluntary associate's experience, but the matters raised are inevitably haphazard and leave many gaps. Teaching is essentially unsystematic and uneven. At the same time the voluntary associate is reacting to his new situation and less able to offer a stable relationship to the client. A further objection to this form of induction is that selection must precede preparation. Any attempt to reject members in the light of attitudes or behaviour revealed during the course is difficult and may be injurious to the clients as well as to the would-be voluntary associates.

But it would be unwise to adopt the type of training used by Teamwork Associates without critical re-appraisal in each new situation. Its courses were planned at a time when every effort was needed to raise the confidence of probation officers in Inner London regarding the potential contribution of voluntary associates. In that climate there was clearly a risk of over-training, but the favourable reaction by both voluntary associates and probation officers, regarding the value of the courses does not suggest that they saw it in that way.

If similar courses were to be run through the country, it is doubtful whether the scale of recruitment in many probation and after-care areas would justify holding them sufficiently frequently to cater for new voluntary associates as and when they came forward. There would seem to be a case for co-operation between areas at regional level, possibly within the framework of NACRO's regional structure. If so it might be necessary to reorganize courses to fit into one or two weekends or a series of day conferences, perhaps on Saturdays. Similarly, there would seem to be scope for conferences for voluntary associates and for their organizers/probation officers to come together regionally to compare experience and to learn from each other.

Selection

The experience of Teamwork Associates suggested that self-selection had merit, but that some formal selection by a panel was also necessary, at the end of the preparation course. It must, however, be admitted that the 'wastage' from courses was high. While all students may be seen as having a valuable learning experience which contributes to public education about offenders and their treatment, there may be a case for further experiment to give an opportunity for self-selection early in the training programmes, followed by more specific preparation for those ready to commit themselves to becoming voluntary associates.

In other areas, especially those where voluntary associates have been recruited from the personal contacts of probation officers, or on the recommendation of people whose opinions are trusted, less formal methods of selection may be applicable. In Inner London and other large urban areas this is unlikely to apply and it is, in any case, arguable that this personal recruitment is too restrictive, drawing only from those sectors of the community from which the probation officers themselves come and from people of whom they 'approve'. If the range of recruitment is broader, the need for formal selection seems to be increased, but herein lies a dilemma: if this process is, at least in part, an attempt to draw in working-class support then it may be argued that the members of that class are less likely to tolerate such selection methods than are their middle-class counterparts. The only escape from the dilemma may be to take greater risks by relaxing formal methods of selection with the possibility that the result will be beneficial in attracting a different kind of candidate but also harmful in allowing through some others who might have been rejected.

The Clients

At the outset of the project, no assumptions were made about the kind of clients who should have been referred to voluntary associates. In retrospect this seems to have been wise. The range of referrals and the expectation of the referring probation officers have constantly extended the scope of the voluntary associate's contribution. This process is still continuing. Thus it would still be unwise to attempt to define the types of clients suitable for such referral.

When the involvement of voluntary associates was being considered following the ACTO Report, there was a tendency to see their contribution as being to help those ex-prisoners who opted voluntarily for after-care. Those subject to statutory licence were usually regarded as the responsibility of the probation officer, little thought having been given to him sharing the case with a voluntary associate. The 1965 Home Office Circular[3] said:

'While this Circular applies primarily to work with discharged offenders who seek after-care voluntarily, much of it also applies to the compulsory supervision of discharged offenders. But the use of volunteers with offenders whose supervision is backed by sanctions, involves special problems and the probation service may prefer to confine any experiment with new methods of using volunteers to voluntary cases in the initial stage.'

In practice, many probation officers working with voluntary associates have involved them with statutory cases. This was also true of Teamworks Associates; and the Youth Resettlement Project was, of course, wholly geared to the needs of those released on statutory licence.

Similarly, it was at first felt that parole was not an appropriate area of work for voluntary associates. Clearly the primary responsibility for supervision of the parolee must rest upon the probation officer but the first report of the Parole Board[4] said:

'The load carried by the Probation and After-Care Service has already been stressed, and in many areas the Service has enlisted the help of volunteers. This is one way in which, with discretion, members of the public without special training, but with the advice of a professional social worker, can help.'

If the inmate who is homeless, without family or friends, or in special need of support, is to be given a fair chance to qualify for parole, then it can be argued that the provision of voluntary associates could be regarded in appropriate cases as a priority.

Any tidy arrangement at an early stage which might have seen the voluntary associate involved with voluntary after-care and the statutory probation officer with statutory after-care would not have accorded with subsequent experience. Many voluntary cases need professional help; many statutory cases seem to need voluntary help, in addition to the official relationship with the probation officer.

In planning Teamwork Associates much thought was given to defining broad categories of client which might be 'suitable' for voluntary associates, e.g. 'the homeless', 'the lonely or socially isolated'. Consideration was given to concentrating on those committed to prison for the first time or perhaps for the second, who seemed to be at a crucial stage, if further recidivism was to be prevented.

In view of the need to obtain sufficient referrals to keep all the voluntary associates in work, any such preconceptions about types of referral

would have been unworkable, and premature. In any case, broad cate-
gorization along the above lines seems rigid and restrictive.

Even after three years' experience any attempt to lay down hard and
fast guidelines for choosing cases would seem hazardous, but experience
so far suggests that it is unwise or unfair to ask a voluntary associate to
cope alone with a client who has serious personal problems. Such a
client requires professional treatment, usually by the probation officer,
though the voluntary associate may be involved as well. A voluntary
associate alone cannot offer the casework (or therapy) needed by the
psychologically disturbed client. Similarly, the voluntary associate may
not be able to cope alone with the inadequate client who is markedly
immature, mentally retarded or psychopathic. Again professional skills
seem to be appropriate.

On the other hand, where a client has few personal problems, or
seems psychologically fairly 'normal', but has serious problems in his
situation, this may be a case where the voluntary associate could help
without necessarily the direct involvement of the probation officer
(though he would still be in the background to advise). For example, a
man who on his discharge from prison has no home to return to and no
family may, as we have seen, be helped by a voluntary associate, and a
man whose family are hostile or unsympathetic towards him on discharge may value the support of a voluntary associate.

Where the client has a combination of personal and situational problems, both a probation officer and a voluntary associate may be needed.
For example, a probation officer trying to help a psychologically disturbed client through individual casework may enlist the help of a
voluntary associate to give companionship or support which is lacking
in the client's situation. In more favourable situations, this companionship or support might have been enlisted from the client's family or
friends. Thus the voluntary associate may be used as a substitute for
the resources available to help the client in a 'normal' situation.

The Role of the Voluntary Associate

Any attempt to be more specific about the selection of clients depends
upon establishing a more detailed definition of the role of the voluntary
associate. Even at the end of a three-year project this was difficult. It
was still developing, but with the benefit of the experience of the project
it is possible to detect various facets of the role. While these are neither
mutually exclusive nor comprehensive they do offer some practical
guidance as to what the voluntary associate has to offer and how it can

be utilized. They are not an exhaustive list; with further experience others may be added, and in any given case, specific ones may be present which do not fit under these more general headings.

For the client who is still in an institution the voluntary associate may be initially a *contact* in the outside community. For the homeless and alienated man he may be their only contact, providing *a link* with 'normality' and demonstrating that the client is not totally rejected or forgotten. As a link the voluntary associate may be able to help him re-establish relationships in the community.

Whether the relationship is established during or after sentence, the voluntary associate may become a *companion*, someone who is willing to enter into a personal relationship and offer acceptance. By so doing he may be able to restore in the client a sense of personal worth in contrast to the profound sense of unworthiness which can result from or be reinforced by his conviction and imprisonment. Frequently the voluntary associate simply described this as being *a friend*, but only occasionally after some time did the relationship merit that name in its fullest sense. More often 'befriending' would have been nearer to the truth, thus acknowledging the frequent imbalance in the relationship, although it can sound patronizing.

The voluntary associate may, as we have noted, become *a supporter*, a source of encouragement and reassurance to the client. This may involve giving direct practical help, though often he will be encouraged by the probation officer to help the client to help himself, thus avoiding undue dependence, if possible. In this way the voluntary associate may be seen as *an enabler*.

So far these facets have had to do with the personal relationship between voluntary associate and client. If, however, the end product is to be re-integration into the community then the voluntary associate may need to be *an introducer*. Some are better placed than others to introduce their clients to their friends or social groups. For a voluntary associate who lacks the appropriate kind of interests and contacts his job may be primarily to give the client support and to help him re-establish confidence in the making of relationships through their own meetings so that he is better equipped to re-establish links in the outside world. For the client who has the ability to do this, the voluntary associate may be a source of support which enables him to 'ride out' the crises of the first few weeks or months after discharge. This can be seen as a way of 'buying time' in which the client who is reasonably capable of re-integration has a chance to do so in his own way, at his own pace.

For the most damaged and alienated client, any prospect of re-integration seems remote. His alienation has gone further than simply being homeless. He has reached a stage where he has withdrawn emotionally from normal life in the outside community. To expect him to make the effort to return to the normal community may be too demanding and could precipitate breakdown, perhaps in the form of further offences as a means of retreating into the safety of prison. It may well be argued that such a client is far too damaged for a voluntary associate to help, but there are occasions when he establishes contact with one (especially in projects which have no probation officer or other professional social workers responsible for referring clients to voluntary associates). The chances of maintaining contact may be poor and similarly 'progress' unlikely, but a voluntary associate, who by accident or design, finds himself trying to cope with a seemingly impossible situation often feels under an obligation to carry on.

If the client is unable to change appreciably, then any improvement in his situation depends upon some change on the part of those with whom he comes into contact. The voluntary associate becomes *a protector* and may try to persuade employers, landladies, social agencies or magistrates to be a little more tolerant and understanding. In these circumstances the voluntary associate can be seen as acting as *a buffer* between client and community.

Some have seen the voluntary associate as *a representative* of the community, but few came from the same local community as their clients. Nor did they feel that the community, local or global, was behind them in their work. Even so, at a conceptional rather than practical level the representative function of the voluntary associate helps to give meaning to the whole operation.

Types of Voluntary Associate for Types of Client

If some voluntary associates prove to be more effective in one facet of the role than in another, then the question to be asked is not what sort of client is suitable for a voluntary associate, but which of them needs someone as a link with the outside world, which needs someone to help to introduce them to individuals or groups, or which needs support of the kind that could be given by an understanding lay person etc?

Once we do this, we begin to postulate a series of roles which although not mutually exclusive are more distinct than just facets of a single role. At this stage a further question emerges. Is it possible that certain sources of recruitment might be able to provide a sort of voluntary associate better able to play one role than those recruited from another source? For example could it be that the working-class voluntary associate for many clients would be better placed to act as *an introducer* than would a middle-class one, (though the experience of the project showed that the latter could sometimes overcome difficulties in playing this role)? Similarly, could it be that the middle-class voluntary associate is better equipped to be *a supporter* and perhaps more acceptable to some clients in this role because he has come to expect help from persons whose background differs appreciably from his own? Certainly where a voluntary associate acts in a protective role, middle-class competence in dealing with agencies and officials clearly pays dividends. This line of thought strongly supports efforts to broaden the range of recruitment: it also has implications for training and selection which might lead to greater diversity and flexibility.

Matching and Classification of Clients

The above discussion may also lead to a more systematic basis for matching. If clients were classified according to their treatment needs it might be possible in consultation with the voluntary associates individually to decide with which sort of need they are best able to help. Pendleton[5] argued that voluntary associates were best used to cope with specific needs rather than in more complex situations. Some sort of pairing could be done, matching type of treatment need with type of voluntary associate according to his preference or suitability.

If we accept the notion of integration or re-integration into the community as the main objective of after-care, two factors seem paramount in planning the rehabilitation of any client: the degree of his alienation from the community; and his capacity for integration or reintegration.

(1) Where imprisonment constitutes only a temporary physical separation from the community and no permanent damage is done to the client's relationships outside, after-care needs may be minimal and of short duration. The involvement of a voluntary associate would seem improbable as the client is likely to have family and friends to assist him.

(2) Where imprisonment has led to some strain or temporary severing of relationships outside, but there is a reasonable prospect of repairing them, the main need may be for the probation officer to mediate, though sometimes a voluntary associate may be a source of background support for the client. (This may also be a case where help for the family during sentence may help to prevent breakdown or pave the way for reconciliation after discharge.)

(3) Where imprisonment, perhaps repeatedly or for a long period, has led to a breakdown of relationships outside, and to an advanced state of alienation, the crucial question may be how far the client is capable of making the effort to integrate or re-integrate into the community and, perhaps, how far he is still an acceptable person to the community. If it seems that there is a chance of a satisfactory re-acceptance, then the voluntary associate, in conjunction with the probation officer, may be a means of aiding re-introduction; if such a process seems remote any attempt to overcome the client's alienation may amount to an intolerable demand upon him. Here the objective may need to be much more limited—to give companionship, support and protection just so long as he can tolerate it.

Evaluation and Co-ordination

If future developments of voluntary associate work are to provide a means of learning, there is a need for more systematic and independent evaluation than it was possible for Teamwork Associates to attempt. Unfortunately efforts to build in research greatly adds to the cost of any project and suitably qualified research workers are not often available. A further problem can arise if those initiating the project fail to understand the technical limitations of much research in the social sciences and thus set too high an expectation of it. But there is a need for a series of experimental projects with built-in research and, again, this can only be done effectively with a measure of central co-ordination and leadership. NACRO may have a key role in this respect.

For the reasons stated, only a few projects could be included in such a research programme; for the rest, it would be essential to give them every opportunity to learn from these examples of 'action research' as they progressed. This process of continuous sharing could be seen as part of a wider network of contacts between projects so that all those involved in their leadership have frequent opportunities for co-operation and for learning from each other. The lack of this so far is to be regretted, but again it is a field where NACRO may be able to facilitate the interchange of experience.

REFERENCES

1. Op. cit., Ch. 3.
2. Op. cit., par. 16.
3. Ibid., par. 3.
4. Report of the Parole Board for 1968 HMSO.
5. Op. cit., par. 198.

CHAPTER 15

SOME IMPLICATIONS FOR THE WIDER
INVOLVEMENT OF THE VOLUNTEER

The Volunteer in Probation and After-Care

For a pilot project, it was necessary to define the boundaries so that the experience gained was fairly intensive. Even so the range of work done by the voluntary associates was constantly extended and it was necessary to revise the initial notions about their role to embrace variations in it.

A point was reached where voluntary associates were in touch with almost all categories of client dealt with by probation officers. Nor were their efforts restricted to individual clients. One team rallied round to give regular support to a young assistant warden temporarily in charge of a hostel. Another team became friends of a new hostel, one woman helping to buy and make soft furnishings, and several of the men regularly visiting the house to provide a link with the local neighbourhood. Others joined in group activities for borstal boys and one woman acted as hostess for an Alcoholics Anonymous group. In Camden the Citizens Advice Bureaux used their workers to interview convicted defendents in the cells of the magistrates' court.

The second Reading Report[1] drew attention to the scope which existed for diversification of the volunteers' efforts. Any attempt to set arbitrary limits on the scope of the volunteers' contribution would be regrettable. The 1965 Home Office Circular[2] said:

'In the present state of knowledge and experience of the subject, it would not be appropriate to delimit the ways in which volunteers can help individual offenders. The help that can be given depends essentially on the capacity of the volunteers to give it, of the probation service to use it, and of the offender to receive it.'

In a fluid and evolving situation, rigid demarcations between one type of volunteer and another could be unnecessarily restrictive, but this can too easily happen where voluntary organizations agree to specialize in particular functions to avoid overlap and to facilitate smooth administration. Sensitivity, flexibility and imagination are needed to recognize the talents of each volunteer and to give him the opportunity to use them where they seem most needed.

Teams of voluntary associates, of the kind established during the project, could become the nucleus for a broader and more dynamic range of voluntary action. 'Action groups' could be established to study local needs and to mobilize resources from the local community. The outcome might be a whole range of new tasks for voluntary action.

A strong case can be made for more volunteers to help families, linked closely with the voluntary associates who would be working with the individual offenders. Developments in this direction call for a substantial investment of professional staff to produce quick results.

Similarly much scope exists for preventive work, especially with young people, for the provision of support services and local ties for hostels, and for public education programmes. These are just a few of the fields where volunteers could fill gaps in the current services.

The Professional Volunteer

Although many of the voluntary associates in the project had professional qualifications that might have been used, the director was reluctant to ask them to give their professional services on the cheap. If they are willing to do so, and providing this does not contravene their professional ethics, much more could be done to use their skills. It requires little imagination to find ways of involving solicitors, publicity experts, research workers and others, especially at headquarters level. Similarly those with technical skills, such as accountants and surveyors, might be assigned to hostel projects.

The Volunteer and the Voluntary Movement

The new generation of volunteers can be seen as reinforcements for the voluntary movement through a variety of voluntary organizations. It will be tragic if, because many of these volunteers have been recruited directly by the Probation and After-Care Service, they fail to find their full place in the wider voluntary movement. This need in no way conflict with their work with their local probation officers.

Many volunteers have no other wish than to be allowed to help the individual client. Clearly it would be foolish and wrong to press them into a much wider range of activities for which they have no appetite. But others who are keen to do more should be given ample opportunities. Whether they also retained contact with clients on a personal basis would be for them to decide, although there can be little doubt that this would keep their feet on the ground and ensure that the clients' interest remained central.

Immense resources within the community to help the offender and his family remain largely untapped. Modest efforts of the sort undertaken by Teamwork Associates are only touching the fringe of these resources. If adequate services are to be provided, and few in the statutory or voluntary services would dare to be complacent about their present state, then much scope still remains to involve more volunteers and give them the fullest opportunity to use their talents.

The Volunteer in the Social Services
But the volunteers in the probation and after-care field must not, indeed cannot, be seen in isolation from those in the mainstream of the social services. Although recent experience in probation and after-care is among the most interesting extensions of the voluntary service, it is only a fraction of the total contribution by the ordinary citizen to the social services. As the project demonstrated, there are substantial practical advantages in drawing voluntary associates from this mainstream of volunteers, especially through go-ahead Councils of Social Service.

Now the Seebohm Report[3] is implemented, the creation of a single local authority social service department will create a new focus for voluntary as well as statutory action. The importance attached in the Report to the full participation of the citizen in the social services could prove to be nothing less than a silent revolution. It will be a major handicap if the Probation and After-Care Service is cut off from the main body of volunteers in the social services.

The Probation and After-Care Service cannot afford to find itself competing with the new social service departments for a share of the resources of the community. Rivalry and duplication can only be wasteful. Probation officers could participate in programmes by social service departments to mobilize community resources including volunteers, some of whom may be assigned subsequently to work with the Probation and After-Care Service for all or part of their voluntary service. If, unhappily, competitive programmes were to be launched, the social service department, with its democratic links in the local community, and with its wider range of attractive opportunities for voluntary service, would be bound to win.

But there is a further and more basic argument for joint action. If after-care is intended to affect the offender's integration or reintegration into the community, the social service department may not only become the main source of the sorts of help which he would need; it may also become the key expression of the community's concern to care for all its citizens including the offender. Unless the ex-prisoner is to be treated as undeserving, preserving the doctrine of less eligibility of the old Poor Law, he is entitled to use the available services of the community like any other citizen.

Taken to its logical conclusion this is an argument for handing over all voluntary after-care to the social service department, through which the full range of statutory and voluntary resources of the community could be made available. Help from that department might well be more acceptable to those ex-prisoners who at present show reluctance to accept any form of after-care. If, however, the extension of parole, or possibly of other forms of statutory after-care, shifts the balance from voluntary to compulsory, such a transfer of responsibility would be inappropriate.

Specialization

There is, however, reason to resist the move towards a 'generic volunteer' in line with the trend towards a single social work profession. The experience of the project showed that voluntary associates were undertaking more demanding and more responsible work than were volunteers in most other fields. Although recruitment, initial interviewing and perhaps one or two introductory talks could usefully be combined, there was a clear need for specialized preparation and selection.

Many volunteers are motivated to help a particular kind of client—the physically handicapped, the aged, or perhaps the offender. By offering specific opportunities there would seem to be better chance of enlisting their help.

There are real dangers in pretending that the offender is no different from other clients. The fact of his criminality cannot be ignored. Even the offender's family faces problems which differ from those of other families in need, in some respects. But neither the offender nor his family, especially when he has completed his sentence, want to be labelled or to be treated as different.

How then can we have our cake and eat it? How can these clients be accepted as members of the community and helped through its normal social services without ignoring their special needs? The answer may lie in using volunteers from the mainstream of the social services, supervised by probation officers, and in providing 'interest groups' where those who have been selected to work with offenders and/or their families can meet to share their specialist experience and to participate in courses and conferences.

An Interim Stage
The reorganization of the social services is not, of course, likely to happen overnight, nor are new departments, faced with complex problems of management and planning, going to be ready to embark upon ambitious programmes to involve the community straight away. Indeed the grand designs of the Seebohm Report for the participation of the citizen might never develop.

Practical plans for volunteers in the probation and after-care field cannot rely upon such an uncertain prospect, but nor can they afford to miss the chance to be involved if and when such radical changes begin. In the meantime, Councils of Social Service may, if they are willing and active, be a means, in some areas, of linking the volunteer working with the offender and/or his family with the mainstream of volunteers, while NACRO could provide the specialist focus for them.

Community Development
In this chapter we have been discussing the ever widening scope for the volunteer, but there is a trend also towards a more spontaneous and informal attempt to mobilize the resources of the community, often within a local neighbourhood, by means of 'community development.' The Seebohm Report recognized its importance and again it is a type of work where the Probation and After-Care Service must be actively involved so that the needs of the offender and/or his family are included.

It could be argued that just as the influence of social casework theory, for a time, led to the individualization of the client in isolation from his environment, so recent development have repeated the same pattern by individualizing the volunteer and abstracting him from the community, by identifying him with the Probation and After-Care Service. The initial efforts by Teamwork Associates to establish teams within corporate bodies in the community was an attempt to avoid this process. But it was an attempt which proved to be unworkable and again the volunteers became individualized. The creation of borough teams, and the maintenance of a corporate voluntary identity were only partly successful in retaining some community links.

If the recruitment of individual volunteers is regarded as an end in itself then opportunities for a fuller community involvement will be missed. If, however, the current projects for the recruiting of volunteers are seen as a first step in building up contacts in the community, a range of new developments may become possible, including, for example, more self help projects and delinquency prevention schemes. Such developments would be complementary to the contribution of the individual volunteer who is beginning to have an established place in the service for the offender and his family.

REFERENCES

1. Op. cit., par. 47.
2. Op. cit., par. 6.
3. Op. cit., Ch. 16.

CHAPTER 16

SOME IMPLICATIONS FOR ORGANIZATIONAL STRUCTURE

In this chapter it is proposed to consider future organizational structure for the voluntary movement in the light of the Teamwork Associates' experience and the changing structure of the statutory social service.

The Teamwork Associates Model
The particular form of organization adopted by Teamwork Associates was chosen after a careful study of the then existing problems of co-operation between the Probation and After-Care Service and the voluntary organizations in Inner London. It represented an attempt to find a middle way between a claim for total independence by the voluntary organization, and total control or absorption by the statutory service. In practice, it proved difficult to maintain this course, without being dominated by the much larger and stronger statutory service. This became especially difficult at the end of the project when charitable funds were running out and it was decided to ask the Probation and After-Care Committee to take over the full financial responsibility (instead of just a part of it). The need for that committee to be satisfied that public funds were being properly spent implied a degree of control which seemed to threaten the separate identity of the voluntary organization. After much discussion it was agreed that the most effective means of counter-balancing the statutory organization was to establish a larger voluntary organization by combining with the Blackfriars Scheme (and possibly other groups later) under the umbrella of NACRO. In this way, the basic model for partnership between statutory and voluntary was preserved with the possibility of its extension. Thus the work described in the report now forms part of the largest voluntary associate body in London.

Discussion regarding future plans prompted the committee and director of the project to clarify what it was that they wished to preserve.

They thought that the project had hit upon a model which on the one hand satisfied the legitimate expectation of the statutory service to co-ordinate overall policy, to supervise the work of voluntary associates, and to contribute to the maintenance of standards of selection and training; and, on the other hand, maintained a separate identity for the voluntary associates, provided a body primarily concerned with their interests, and a means by which their views could be conveyed to the statutory service. It was felt that voluntary associates should not become second-class citizens of the statutory service, but full members of their own organization. Nor should they be seen as pale shadows of the probation officers, which seems a real risk if they become over-identified with the Probation and After-Care Service. It was also thought that in a complex situation where the statutory service had conflicting demands upon its resources, and problems in defining priorities, the voluntary organizations had been able to pursue clearly defined goals with single-mindedness, enjoying a necessary measure of freedom to experiment, and sometimes to make mistakes.

Applying the Model Elsewhere
But the application of this model in other situations, and at a different point in time, must be examined critically. Outside large urban areas, the number of voluntary associates needed by any one Probation and After-Care Service would not justify the cost of creating a separate voluntary organization of the Teamwork Associates kind. The over-heads in administering a properly constituted company limited by guar-antee, the preparation of separate accounts and so on, would not be warranted. Nor would the secondment of full-time staff seem appro-priate. It might be, and frequently is, more feasible to use several pro-bation officers, each giving a portion of their time. But the possibility of several areas combining to sponsor a joint voluntary associate project could prove to be a more effective solution and would justify the expense entailed. Unless this is considered, efficient management of volunteers may be best undertaken by the Probation and After-Care Service itself (except perhaps in the largest cities). Not surprisingly this is the model which has been adopted most frequently outside London. But it need not exclude the provision of a means by which volunteers can come together under their own auspices to discuss their work and to express their views. During the discussions regarding the future work in Inner London, the creation of an 'association' for volunteers and run by volun-teers was seriously considered. Although it was not selected as a future

model, it may have merit in other areas. Volunteers might be invited to form their own local association electing their own committee and officers (along similar lines to professional associations). Opportunity for these local associations to come together for conferences might be facilitated by NACRO regional organizers.

Devising a Model for a More Complex Future
However, any attempt to devise an organizational structure for the future must take account of the changing structure of the statutory service, which we discussed in the last chapter. If the argument for tying in volunteers in the probation and after-care field with others in the mainstream of social work is accepted, then a more complex organizational structure will be needed. It will no longer be adequate simply to define the relationship between the Probation and After-Care Service and its voluntary partners. In fact, at least four parties seem to be involved (apart from the clients): the Probation and After-Care Service, the voluntary organizations, the local authority social service department and NACRO.

The form of co-operation between these bodies is complex, and must vary accordingly to the nature of the area. Until the future relationship between the local authority social service department and the Probation and After-Care Service has been clarified, it may be premature to consider the matter further.

The Pioneering Role of the Voluntary Organization
It is a paradox that voluntary organizations which in all fields of social service have been pioneers, tend, once established, to become conservative and wedded to their own traditions. At any one time a minority of them are fulfilling this pioneering role while the majority seem to lag behind.

In after-care, many of the older voluntary organizations were slow to adjust to the radical changes following the ACTO Report. A new generation of projects sprang up. Now a further period of change is anticipated with perhaps even more radical implications. The crucial question is whether the present generation of voluntary organizations will follow the example of their predecessors and be largely superseded, or whether there is the willingness to accept change which may upset established attitudes and practices.

If the social services are seen as a partnership between statutory and voluntary organizations, and if the former are radically restructured, a compelling case can be made for doing the same to the latter. It has been said that a Seebohm Report is needed for the voluntary organizations. This may well be so, but they cannot afford to wait for this, or allow events to overtake them, before facing up to the painful need for change.

CHAPTER 17

SOME IMPLICATIONS FOR PROBATION
OFFICERS

Finally some consideration is needed regarding the ways in which probation officers are affected by the increased use of volunteers. The same points may be relevant to other professional social workers in fields where volunteers play an increasingly large part.

The Changing Attitude of the Probation Officer
During the three years of the project, it was gratifying to observe the gradual change in the attitude of probation officers towards volunteers. Initial reluctance to refer work to them has declined, and there is a greater willingness to involve them in long-term relationships with clients. There has been a tendency to use voluntary associates in a variety of roles, some of which require a measure of understanding and skill which tends to encroach upon work which might previously have been reserved for the probation officer.

The Changing Role of the Probation Officer
If this process continues, and the number of volunteers greatly increases, it will have implications for the role of the probation officer, involving the acquisition of new responsibilities and the relinquishing of others. Already some have begun to develop skills in the preparation and supervision of volunteers. These skills have been acquired by trial and error, but this need not be so in the future. Enough is now known to give probation officers who are to be assigned to such duties a short course of inservice training.

But it is not only those officers undertaking these specialist duties whose roles are affected. Whenever a probation officer refers a case to a volunteer with a view to establishing a long-term relationship, his own role changes (see p. 28). If a proportion of cases are to be referred to volunteers or to other agencies, it is necessary for the diagnosis and treatment planning to be rapid and efficient. In those situations where the probation officer retains contact with a view to doing individual casework there is a chance to amend the treatment plans as his assessment is modified, but where early referral is made, errors are more difficult to correct.

In those cases referred to volunteers, officers will need to be taught appropriate methods of 'supervision' (a skill at present only to be expected of senior or tutor officers), and to recognize how this differs from the supervision of probation officers.

In future much more of the probation officer's time may be spent in diagnosis and facilitating 'treatment' by linking the clients with resources in the community. This will have implications for the maintenance of standards of confidentiality, and some probation officers may need to be more open in discussion with non-professionals.

Defining the Boundary between the Professional and the Volunteer
Any attempt to define a rigid boundary between the roles of the professionals and the volunteers cannot be sustained. As the latter are involved in new ways, so that boundary shifts.

But just as it is natural that probation officers should feel apprehensive of having their professional skills 'stolen', so it is also natural for volunteers to want to equip themselves as effectively as possible to help their clients. Some do not feel the need to do this, or would not benefit from it, and in some roles it would clearly be unhelpful or maybe harmful. But others, including many who are professional in their own field, automatically search after a level of understanding and skill which some might think necessary only for the professional. They do not see this as incompatible with their voluntary or amateur status.

The professional social workers, including the probation officer, must not, indeed cannot, claim a monopoly of casework skills. On the other hand half-learned skills in inexperienced hands and without professional supervision can be dangerous. But this is not an argument for depriving all volunteers, in all circumstances, of some measure of casework training. One of the most vital functions of the professional social worker in future could be in 'exporting' their skills so that a wide range of people in the community become better able to help their fellows. This process is already taking place. Training for clergy in counselling, for marriage-guidance counsellors and for some Samaritan workers, already prepares them for work undertaken elsewhere by professional social workers. Pilot projects such as the Blackfriars Family Counselling Project, have done much to demonstrate how carefully selected, prepared and supervised volunteers can provide a service in place of the professional social worker.

Significantly perhaps, it is psychiatrists with their roots in a more secure profession, who have been more ready to encourage the skilled use of volunteers than have professional social workers, who seem more vulnerable. But given high standards of professional practice, they have little cause to fear that the distinction between themselves and the volunteers will be lost. If professional social workers have frequent opportunities to 'recharge their batteries' through in-service training courses, they could be a perpetual source for educating and training volunteers to comparatively high standards.

This process does not, of course, apply purely to volunteers. In prison the need to help the discipline officers to become more skilled in helping the inmate is a challenge to the prison welfare officers. The participation of the police in Juvenile Liaison Schemes presents a similar need. This educational process implies a reversal of the trends of the past 40 years during which professional social workers have often tended to take away responsibility from lay people.

The Leadership Role of the Probation Officer
This discussion may well be worrying to some probation officers and to some other professional social workers, either because they fear that the natural spontaneity of the volunteers is being destroyed and replaced by a quasi-professionalism or because they are unwilling to contemplate the involvement of semi-skilled workers. This can be seen as undermining the hard-fought battle to establish professional social work standards by putting the clock back. But in fact the developments anticipated demand of the professionals a higher standard of competence and skill, and would be likely to lead to enhanced status and much greater need for their services.

Many volunteers will continue to operate in a relatively unskilled way and certainly this was true for nearly all the voluntary associates during the project. For many clients this may be the appropriate sort of help. But other volunteers are likely to become increasingly skilled and in social services starved of adequate trained manpower it would be contrary to the interests of the client to restrict such volunteers.

Recent developments have created the possibility of the active participation of many more citizens, formally and informally, in the social services. Each must be encouraged to equip himself to play his most effective part. In an age of improved education, when many volunteers are drawn from other professional fields, they will expect the opportunity to develop their voluntary service to a high level of competence. To this end the professional social worker has a vital role in education and leadership.

APPENDIX

Teamwork Associates

Preparation Course for Voluntary Associates

Week

1. (a) The Offender and the Community
       An Assistant Principal Probation Officer
   (b) Small Groups: General Discussion

2. (a) Prison and its Purpose
       A Prison Governor
   (b) Small Groups: Case Study

   Visits to prison during the week.

3. (a) Small Groups: Discussion on Visits
   (b) Some Ways in which Institutions Affect People
       A Senior Probation Officer

4. (a) The Prisoner and his Family
       A Senior Probation Officer
   (b) Small Groups: Case Study

5. Discussion Panel on After-Care
       A Senior Probation Officer dealing with after-care for the homeless
       A Senior Probation Officer dealing with after-care for those with homes
       A Prison Welfare Officer

6. (a) The Role of the Voluntary Associate
       The Director, Teamwork Associates
   (b) Discussion Panel with Experienced Voluntary Associates

7. (a) Small Groups: Discussion with Experienced Voluntary Associates
   (b) Course Review

TABLE A

Voluntary Associates in each Borough Team and the Youth Resettlement Project as at July 1969

Camden	16
Greenwich	11
Islington	14
Kensington and Chelsea	18
Lambeth	8
Lewisham	11
Southwark	12
Tower Hamlets	10
Wandsworth	8
Westminster	9
Youth Resettlement Project	38
Total	155
Withdrawals	20
Grand Total	175

TABLE B

Date of Commencement, Duration and Membership of Preparation Courses

Course Number	Starting Dates	Length in Weeks	Total Enrolled	For Teamwork Associates	For Other After-Care Organiza-tions	Applica-tions Made	Applica-tions Accepted
1	16.3.66	—	3	3	—	3	2
2	8.6.66	8	5	4	1	3	3
3	14.9.66	12	23	20	3	10	8
4	10.1.67	11	22	12	10	6	5
5	28.3.67	12	20	20	—	6	4
6	6.4.67	12	20	20	—	5	2
7	25.4.67	8	31	27	4	12	10
8	13.9.67	8	36	34	2	21	17
9	17.10.67	6	20	20	—	7	6
10	1.2.68	7	27	21	6	11	10
11	5.2.68	7	35	30	5	21	19
12	6.5.68	7	38	31	7	17	14
13	9.5.68	8	30	30	—	17	14
14	9.10.68	7	25	23	2	16	13
15	11.2.69	7	26	21	5	14	11

Youth Resettlement Project

1	3.10.68	9	32	32	—	18	15
2	8.1.69	8	16	16	—	6	5
3	15.4.69	8	25	25	—	11	8
	Totals	—	434	389	45	204	166

A further 7 voluntary associates were trained directly by their local probation officers and 2 were transferred from other probation and after-care areas.

TABLE C

*Referrals to Borough Teams and to the Youth
Resettlement Project Subdivided for Each of
the Three Years*

Team	1.6.66—31.5.67	1.6.67—31.5.68	1.6.68—31.5.69	Totals
Camden	—	2	26	28
Greenwich	—	10	10	20
Islington	3	6	11	20
Kensington & Chelsea	2	6	25	33
Lewisham	—	8	15	23
Lambeth	1	22	8	31
Southwark	2	6	6	14
Tower Hamlets	—	11	6	17
Wandsworth	—	2	8	10
Westminster	5	6	2	13
Youth Resettlement Project	—	—	28	28
	13	79	145	237

TABLE D

Type of Client (At Times of Referral)

Prisoner	75
Ex-prisoner	35
Prisoner and his family	3
Prisoner's family	30
Borstal boy or girl	39
Detention centre boy	1
Ex-borstal boy or girl	10
Ex-detention centre boy	1
Probationer	30
Ex-probationer	3
Probationer and his family	1
Conditional discharge	2
Suspended sentence	1
Matrimonial case	3
Affiliation proceeding case	1
Offender's friend	2
	237

TABLE E

Sources from which Prisoners and Others in Institutions were Referred

Prisons		Borstals	
Pentonville	20	Rochester	12
Shepton Mallet	10	Feltham	11
Wormwood Scrubs	7	Dover	4
Wandsworth	7	Portland	4
Grendon Underwood	6	Holloway (borstal wing)	3
Springhill	5	Gaynes Hall	1
Brixton	3	Hollesley Bay	1
Chelmsford	3	Morton Hall	1
Ford	3	Onley	1
Camp Hill	2	Market Drayton	1
Blundeston	2		39
Albany	1		
Eastchurch	1	*Other Institutions*	
Lewes	1	Goudhurst Detention Centre	1
Maidstone	1	St Margaret Remand Home, Sydenham	1
Parkhurst	1	Blantyre House Remand Centre	1
Preston	1		
Overseas	1		
	75		3

TABLE F

Principal Current Offence of Clients

i. *Offences Against the Person*
   1. Violence against the person — 14
   2. Sexual offences — 19
ii. *Offences against Property*
   3. Breaking offences — 27
   4. Robbery — 8
   5. Thefts and frauds — 83
   6. Receiving — 3
   7. Malicious damage — 4
iii. *Miscellaneous*
   8. Other offences — 26
Not known — 17
Non-offenders — 36

237

TABLE G

*Voluntary Prison After-Care by the Inner London Probation
and After-Care Service, 1967*

Length of Contact	Males	Cases in which a Volunteer Assisted	Females	Cases in which a Volunteer Assisted
One interview only	1,508	195	28	3
Less than 1 month	416	62	12	2
Over 1 but under 2 months	187	24	5	1
Over 2 but under 3 months	235	42	3	—
Over 3 but under 4 months	141	31	4	1
Over 4 but under 5 months	112	22	4	1
Over 5 but under 6 months	124	19	2	—
Over 6 months	554	127	26	5
Total	3,277	522	84	13

INDEX